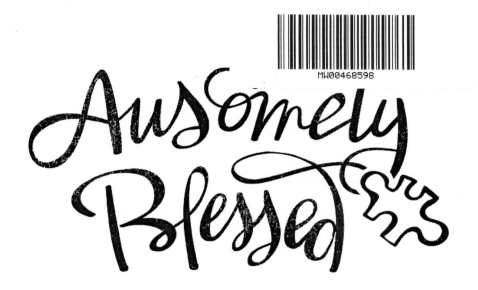

Au·some·ly Bless·ed

//Def. // ...the invoking of God's favor upon a person
through an intellectual or developmental
disability, causing or inducing awe;
inspiring an overwhelming feeling of
reverence and admiration//

{ Source: *God's Dictionary* }

BETH FRANK
and Others

Contents

Dedication

To Luci Frank for helping me see the world in a whole new way and giving me a front row seat to God's grace and everyday miracles. You are my star!

To Ryan, just thank you. Thanks for loving Jesus. Thanks for loving me. Thanks for loving our girls and showing them Jesus through your life. Thanks for believing in me. Thanks for encouraging me. Thanks for being my best friend. Thanks for being you. I crazy love everything about you!

To Mom and Dad, your help, patience, and guidance in my life is immeasurable and I thank God for you every day, literally multiple times a day. I couldn't begin to attempt to thank you for all the ways you have made my life great, but I do thank you for the best thing: thank you for introducing me to Jesus and faithfully teaching me his ways.

To Perry and Judy, thank you for being my second set of parents. I am blessed by you, blessed by your prayers, blessed by your love, blessed by your encouragement, and blessed to call you family.

To Abby, you know what I'm thinking before I say it. You understand and tell me when my crazy is showing! You are a therapist and you are my sister. God knew I would need a sister-therapist, LOL! Seriously, you have helped me immeasurably by loving me and Luci unconditionally and always being a sounding board and listening ear. I find constant comfort in the fact that my sister and best friend always has my back."

To Kristy, you were the first person I told a small part of the idea God gave me and I don't know if I would have had the courage to do this if you hadn't spoken life about this right from the start. #youraisemeup ;)

To each person who submitted a story for the "We Love Luci" chapters. You really are our people! I am amazed as I think about the support system that God has built around Luci. Each and every one of you is an answer to prayer, and I am so grateful for the part you have played in Luci's story. It is no small thing that you have reached out to us, become friends with our girl, and showed us concern and care. The Frank family is forever grateful to each one of you. Go team Luci!

And to Jesus, thank you for calling me, thank you for equipping me, and thank you for loving me and forgiving me as I try, mess up, and try again. This is ultimately for you as a testament to the miracle you worked in a scared and self-centered mom. Thank you for never giving up on me.

introduction

Ausome Blessings in Clay Jars

"Now we have this treasure in clay jars, so that this extraordinary power may be from God and not from us. We are pressured in every way but not crushed; we are perplexed but not in despair; we are persecuted but not abandoned; we are struck down but not destroyed." — 2 Corinthians 4:7-9

HOW CAN LIVING WITH A disability be a blessing? Where is the blessing in hundreds of doctor visits? Where is the silver lining in fighting about coverage with insurance? How can I see greatness when those around me see less than? Where is the joy and freedom of abundant life, when everyday tasks are just plain hard? For those of us in the trenches of life with a person with an intellectual or developmental disability, it is hard to live with the perspective of great blessing and favor. In the world's economy we have been dealt a difficult hand, and our life can seem to be marginalized because we don't meet the criteria for greatness. But what if we stopped looking for blessing in ease, comfort, and perfection? What if we opened our eyes to the treasures right in front of us in clay jars? In God's economy the ways that he can shower his children with blessings are limitless. He has given us gifts in earthen vessels, and we have to be willing to open them.

I am a frequent flyer and unfortunately I am also an anxious flyer. These two facts do not mix well. I have to travel about once a month for work. And although I have prayed and fasted about my fear of flying, many times my anxiety gets the best of me. Turbulence is my nemesis. I can be prayed up and praised up but as soon as the plane starts to bounce around like a small toy at 32,000 feet, my heart drops to my toes. In my most desperate moments, when I am fighting a full-blown panic attack, I will close my eyes and picture the plane flying and the hand of God right beneath it. I know that nothing touches me unless he deems it for my good and his glory. I also will close my eyes and sing that old hymn "grace, grace, God's grace, grace that is greater than all my sins." There is something about focusing on God's grace that can quickly put everything else into perspective. I don't deserve the life I live, I don't deserve to be flying off somewhere to do ministry, I don't deserve the beautiful family that he has given me, and I certainly don't deserve a forever home with him in heaven. On this last flight though, a new thought crept into my mind as we were going through an extended period of turbulence, i.e. torture! I thought to myself, *you like roller coasters and Luci LOVES them, so keep your eyes closed, pretend this is a rollercoaster, and enjoy the turbulence.* It was at this point that I realized that I was actually certifiably crazy! But you know what? It worked! I made it my goal to enjoy the bumps along the way and not to fear them, and my entire body felt the peace from the change in my perspective.

I know that the premise for this book sounds crazy! Blessings from a special needs diagnosis and peace from pain—that makes no earthly sense, but neither does putting treasure in jars of clay. My goal for this book is to encourage those living life with a person with a physical or intellectual disability. No, I don't want you to close your eyes and pretend that it never happened, but I do want you to close your eyes and say "grace, grace, God's grace." He has placed so many blessings right in our paths, and some of them are ausome jars of clay! Yes, we will face lots of bumps along the way—"We are pressured in every way but not crushed; we are perplexed but not in despair; we are persecuted but not abandoned; we are struck down but not destroyed"—but it's all to show the extraordinary power of God at work! We can enjoy the bumps knowing that we are living an ausomely blessed life right smack dab in the middle of God's palm!

Over the last decade I have been on a journey with Jesus, during which he has shifted my mindset in this way. My journey from first hearing my daughter Luci's diagnosis to accepting her diagnosis to living in the reality of the blessing of her diagnosis was a long one—ashamedly, a very long one. But it's a story of God taking me full circle to realize that not all blessings come in the way we expect them.

Only God could have taken an incredibly anxious, fearful, first-time mom and turn her into someone who faced the future with peace and certainty. Peace and certainty in knowing that God is writing Luci's story and he defines who she is and how she will bring him glory.

I now see on a daily basis how God is writing our story with ausome opportunities, ausome influence, ausome everyday miracles, ausome innocence, ausome potential, and ausome love. It's only by letting go of the pen and trusting his hand to write the story that has enabled him to bring me full circle into the ausomely blessed life he has for me.

Once I came to realize that we were more than just okay, we were blessed, I wanted other families with specially-abled children to realize the same thing. Life with these kiddos is a blessing—in James the Bible says, every good and perfect gift comes from above, and Luci and all these individuals are most definitely good and perfect gifts!

9

God gave me the idea for this book, a book that would be a collaboration of different ministry friends each sharing their unique viewpoint of how life with a disability can be one of blessing and favor. Each of these authors has a unique perspective and a passion to encourage those who have been affected by an intellectual or developmental disability. I think you will appreciate the heart behind their words as they seek to practically love and support special needs families and their children.

While I was working on the content for this book, I realized that our family, like so many other families that have ausome kiddos, has so many God stories of everyday miracles. I asked my family and friends to share some of their favorite Luci stories. I have dedicated two chapters to this, not to bring attention to us, but to testify to the greatness of God. He has built a community of love around our daughter, and we are continually seeing his extraordinary power in spite of being just jars of clay.

My prayer is that you receive inspiration as well as practical help from the pages of this book. May you be blessed and your heart encouraged by all that is possible when God decides to bless ausomely!

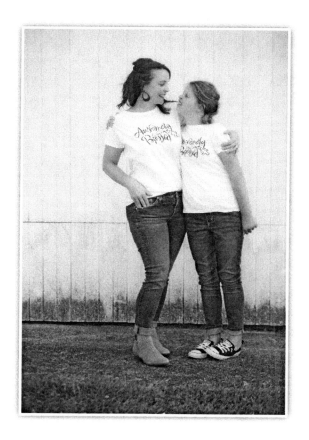

chapter 1

Ausome Love

by Beth Frank

JESUS' HEART FOR THE LEAST of these is, to me, one of the most beautiful parts of scripture. Our God loves and is near to the weak and distressed. In the New Testament there are many stories of Jesus healing and reaching out to the outcasts of society. The people who were invisible to their communities, Jesus stops and sees them, really sees them, touches them, and heals them physically and emotionally. Can you imagine, being blind for your entire life, helpless and almost invisible to society, and one day a stranger stops in front of you?! He speaks to you and touches you! You aren't ever touched in a loving way; then this stranger touches your eyes and as sight comes to your eyes for the very first time, your eyes lock on his and the first sight you see is indescribable love coming from the one who loves you most. The story in Luke 18 brings tears to my eyes every time I read it. God's love and special care for individuals with a disability is displayed again and again throughout scripture. We can take hope and comfort knowing that God seeks out and has a deep love for those who are ausomely blessed.

Let me introduce myself. My name is Beth, and this is the part of my story where ausome love found me.

When I was younger, I had a very definite idea of how my story would go, and when the storyline of my life started taking a turn that I never intended, I had a hard time seeing the beauty in it. If we have accepted Jesus as our savior, we understand the Biblical truth that right now there is an amazing story being written—the story of God's redemption of his creation through Jesus his son. Psalm 111:9 says, "He sent redemption to his people; he has commanded his covenant forever. Holy and awesome is his name." We can all easily agree with that and see the amazing beauty of that story. But sometimes, it's how he writes our own stories in the scheme of that larger narrative that trips us up.

Growing up I had plans and some serious goals. I took for granted that I would marry prince charming (that actually happened) and we would have a couple of typical children and that life would be one fabulous adventure! I grew up as a pastor's child, so I knew to expect that there would be bumps along the way and not everything would be blissfully perfect, but I didn't realize then what I've learned now, and that is the truth that God is writing my story with his pen. Psalm 139:16 says, "Your eyes saw my unformed body; all the days ordained for me were written in your book before one of them came to be." I can embrace the life he has called me to or I can constantly run in another direction, losing opportunities to give him glory through my circumstances.

When you get to be an adult, it's quite surprising to realize there are many things you have no control over. A lot of times we only can control our responses to our situations. In the book *Chase the Lion*, Mark Batterson says, "Inciting incidents come in two basic varieties: things that happen to you that you cannot control and things you make happen that you can control. Of course, even if something is out of your control, you still control your reaction. You might not be responsible, but you are response-able. And it's the ability to choose your response that will likely determine your destiny."

You see we can choose to live surrendered lives that daily give God control. Basically we are living with our hands held up, opened-palmed with the things we hold most dear in this world: our spouse, our children, our dreams, our goals, our money, and then make decisions that honor God in the circumstances he has placed us in. Living in surrender like this changes our perspective. Living like this is how God can show up loving in our situations where we don't see the disease, failure, setback, or diagnosis, but we see, blessing, grace, and mercy.

My daughter Luci Frank came into the world on October 16, 2004. Luci was my miracle baby from the beginning. She was the answer to years of praying for a baby and arrived a month early, but seemed to be in perfect health. The storyline I was writing was slightly off track at this point, but with her arrival, I knew that we could make up for lost time! Her infancy was filled with joy and wonder as my husband Ryan and I settled into the role of parents. As I look back now, I see the warning signs started early, but as a first-time mom, I was in love with motherhood and my sweet baby girl and was blissfully unaware of the struggle to come.

As Luci approached two and her vocabulary seemed to be lagging behind others her age, we immediately began speech therapy and had preliminary testing done by specialists in Indy. Everyone assured me that all would be well with Luci. They said she was a bright girl and that in time she would catch up, but in my heart, I felt that something was wrong, seriously wrong.

I was panicked, trying to figure out what I could do to help my little girl and trying to figure out what could be the problem. Over the next few years we met with multiple doctors and therapists, sought treatment through traditional and nontraditional therapies, tried diets and supplements, and tried traditional preschool as well as a special needs preschool. It was constantly on my mind day or night and my burden to help Luci stole my peace and Joy. I cried out to God like never before and clung to verses like Romans 8:28, which says, "We know that all things work together for the good of those who love God: those who are called according to His purpose."

It was during this time that God spoke to my spirit in a very profound way. I really had never experienced anything like it up until that point. At my most panicked times, at the times when I didn't know which direction to go, at the times when it didn't seem we were making any progress at all, he would whisper to my spirit, "Everything will be okay. I love Luci and everything is okay." I clung to that promise when nothing around me seemed to support that. My greatest fear was that Luci would be diagnosed with autism or have a significant cognitive impairment or that she would not be able to communicate easily for years to come.

I remember sometime during those early years, my sister Abby, who is a therapist and was working in the social services field, told me about a client. (Abby never shares specifics about her clients). She had met someone who didn't start to speak until around age nine. At that time in my life I couldn't even imagine that being our story. God had promised me that everything was okay, and that wasn't our story. No, my little girl would speak much sooner than that. I couldn't bear to wait to have a conversation with Luci till she was nine—that was unthinkable.

In our world today it's easy to believe that if something is wrong with you health-wise, you can go to a doctor and they can tell you what's wrong and then fix it. That has certainly not been the case for me in my adult life! Our brain is a complex organ that modern medicine still knows shockingly little about. An autism diagnosis doesn't just come overnight and it has taken years to be able to tell how serious Luci's case is. Even now, it's hard to tell exactly what her future will look like and what she will be able to do.

Luci was diagnosed with autism. She does have a cognitive impairment and she didn't really start talking in sentences until around eight or nine years old—my greatest fears were realized. But when we finally made it to that point, I realized that I was okay and that Luci was okay. I also realized that the promise God had given me about how we would be okay had more to do with me than with her. The healing that I had been praying for had more to do with me and my heart than with the physical needs of Luci. My heart had needed a spiritual healing. I came to the realization that Luci had been okay all along and it was me who needed to be okay with her. God was working out that promise in my life and bringing my heart complete peace about life with autism. He was bringing me full circle. We were living in the reality of what I had been so fearful about all those years earlier, but it was okay. God had kept his promise to me.

How did God bring me to this place? So far I have given you a snapshot of our outward journey, but the journey that God took my heart through during that time was just as profound. Sadly I refer to Luci's early years as my dark years. I would tell Ryan that I could never feel complete joy again because of what Luci was going through. When your kids are born, you have dreams for them, plans for the things you want to do with them, expectations of how things will be. It seemed as if daily I would go through the realization of another dream dying. I wouldn't be having conversations with my little girl anytime soon. Going to the store and shopping together would probably be something she never enjoyed. Hugs and kisses from her would be very rare. Sharing simple pleasures like reading a book together or taking a bike ride would be difficult. Friends would be few and far between for my girl. School wouldn't look anything like what we had thought. I could go on and on. It was because of the death of these dreams that everything but getting help for Luci went dark for me. I became very secluded. I really couldn't identify with the moms around me because my reality was vastly different from theirs. That promise that Luci would be okay became very dim.

I read a story a few years ago by Emily Kingsley titled "Welcome to Holland" that captured me immediately. The story really does a good job explaining the myriad of feelings one experiences when finding out you will be parenting a child with a disability.

Welcome to Holland

When you're going to have a baby, it's like planning a fabulous vacation trip to Italy. You buy a bunch of guide books and make your wonderful plans. The Coliseum. Michelangelo's David. The gondolas in Venice. You may learn some handy phrases in Italian. It's all very exciting. After months of eager anticipation, the day finally arrives. You pack your bags and off you go. Several hours later, the plane lands. The stewardess comes in and says, "Welcome to Holland."

"Holland?!" you say. "What do you mean Holland? I signed up for Italy! I'm supposed to be in Italy. All my life I've dreamed of going to Italy." But there's been a change in the flight plan. They've landed in Holland and there you must stay.

The important thing is that they haven't taken you to a horrible, disgusting, filthy place, full of pestilence, famine, and disease. It's just a different place. So you must go out and buy new guide books. And you must learn a whole new language. And you will meet a whole new group of people you would never have met.

It's just a different place. It's slower-paced than Italy, less flashy than Italy. But after you've been there for a while and you catch your breath, you look around ... and you begin to notice that Holland has windmills ... and Holland has tulips. Holland even has Rembrandts.

But everyone you know is busy coming and going from Italy, and they're all bragging about what a wonderful time they had there. And for the rest of your life, you will say, "Yes, that's where I was supposed to go. That's what I had planned."

And the pain of that will never go away because the loss of that dream is a very significant loss. But if you spend your life mourning the fact that you didn't get to Italy, you may never be free to enjoy the very special, the very lovely things about Holland.

Time went on and I began to adjust to our new reality. Life skills, IEP, ABA, insurance pre-certification, waiver, biomedical, and gluten free all became my new normal. Through it all Luci was a trooper and I loved her more and more each day and was willing to fight for her more and more each day, but honestly, the days were hard, and they were long, and sometimes they were scary because the future was so uncertain. During this time I had one of my worst parenting moments *ever* along with the most audible God moment. God spoke to me in a direct way. He used our then eight-year-old Luci to speak straight from heaven to my heart. I hesitate to share this story because it is not my proudest moment and came in one of the most difficult seasons of my life, but God has been working in my heart that Romans 8:28 is all about the good times and the bad ones. He is working to make all things good for his glory. He is redeeming my dark times for my good and his glory. I share this story hoping that it will bring him glory and give encouragement that the heart of a special needs child is so close to the heart of God.

When our Luci was around six years old, my husband and I started having serious reservations about how well our public school was doing at addressing her unique needs. We always hear how early intervention is key and I was feeling the pressure that it was now or never, we needed to do something radical. Luci was still pretty non-verbal and had a serious elopement issue. She had made it actually outside of her school building (that sat right off a very busy highway) not once, but twice that school year. We prayed and the Lord opened many doors for her to be able to attend an amazing school/therapy facility about an hour from our home. This was a huge sacrifice for our family in time and finances. My second daughter was around eighteen months old and we downsized to a Mini Cooper to save on gas. I would load both girls up every morning at seven to start the hour trip to school. I will never forget looking in my rearview mirror and seeing both of their car seats squeezed into the back of that Mini Cooper. Family togetherness! My family really stepped up to help us during this time and it was a true blessing. Ryan's dad religiously picked Luci up every Wednesday and my grandma would also pick Luci up occasionally.

During our first summer attending this new school/therapy, Luci had her first of only four complete meltdowns. I still don't know what caused these. I think that it had something to do with a medication that she was on at the time. These meltdowns were epic, not anything like a meltdown we had experienced before. They came out of the blue, and she could not be calmed in anyway.

Her first was with Ryan and me, while we were stuck in a traffic jam on the interstate. I was truly afraid that she was going to get out of the car and hurt herself or her sister badly. Navigating something like this was out of my wheelhouse. We had never experienced behavior like this with Luci before, and I was unsure how to help her. She was so tormented. I held her to keep her in the car and keep her from hurting herself. After the meltdown we were both covered in sweat and tears. I immediately made contact with her doctor who said it was a summer fit because she had got out of her routine on vacation. I knew better, but thought that since it hadn't happened again that maybe it was just some random thing that Luci had gotten upset about.

Fast forward a month and Luci was back to attending therapy every day, having had no more bizarre behavior. I was handling a work event and my grandma had offered to pick Luci up from school. My cell phone rang when my grandma should have been about halfway home with Luci. My heart sank before I even heard my grandma's voice, because I could hear Luci screaming in the background. Luci was having a meltdown in the back of my grandma's car, and I was at least thirty minutes away. My grandma had pulled over, but she feared that Luci would get out of the car. She was trying to climb into the front seat and grab the steering wheel. My grandma is mighty in spirit but mini in frame. I knew she would be no match for Luci. I grabbed my keys and headed out the door telling my grandma I would be there as soon as I could.

When I arrived, there was a police car there with the lights on. It still makes me cry to think about that scene. My grandma was bawling her eyes out because she didn't know what to do and Luci was being restrained in the backseat of the car while the officers tried to calm her down. Her hair was a rat's nest from all her struggles; her face was beat red and covered in tears. She was calming down and when she saw me, she just started to cry a broken cry that broke my heart.

I know that my Grandma did the right thing. She called the police because she was so scared that she wouldn't be able to keep Luci safe, but at the time I was so unnerved by the sight of a police officer holding my little girl in her seat.

After speaking with the officers, I put Luci into my car and we started home. I really was at the end of my strength. I had been taking my sweet little girl to specialists since she was eighteen months old. We had tried therapies, medication, bio-medical treatment, special diets, and now intensive ABA. I had read every book on autism that I could get my hands on, and talked with other parents to try to learn from them. All of this without much success for Luci and without much change in her verbal skills or behavior and I was *tired*! This momma had gone on her own strength for far too long.

I am so ashamed to tell you what I did in those moments. I cried and yelled. Not really to Luci—it was more against God. I didn't think that I could handle having Luci. I felt like I wasn't qualified in any way to be her mommy. I was angry that God had allowed this to happen. I asked Luci, "Where do you want to live?" I wasn't really expecting a response; she didn't talk much at all beyond the few words she had in her repertoire. It was more a question to God, like, "Who else can do this?" Because at that moment, I am ashamed to say that it only felt like a burden that I had carried way too long. As I looked in the rearview mirror and said again to Luci, "I don't know how I am going to do this. Where do you want to live?"

She looked right at me and as clear as day said, "Heaven."

The hair on the back of my neck stood straight up. The atmosphere in the car changed immediately, and I felt God's presence envelop Luci and me. He had spoken to me directly through my little girl. That one simple word "heaven" changed everything. I gained a new perspective. God had a plan for Luci and he loved her so much. Life was difficult for her and her heart yearns for a day when she will be understood by everyone and be with the one who understands her now. With that one word spoken, I lost all of my anger and frustration and realized that I was blessed to have Luci. With that one word spoken, my heart was changed to know that God was near and he was looking after Luci and I could just stop all the scrambling and frantic attempts to make everything okay, because everything *was* okay. The God of the universe showed up in my car on a country road in Indiana to speak through a little girl in a powerful way. Heaven is indeed near in these special kiddos that are so loved by our God.

One of my biggest regrets in life is that I did not accept the beautiful little girl that God had given me sooner. I loved her always, but I didn't enjoy her like I should have. I needed to enter her world instead of continually trying to get her to enter mine. I believe that when a child is diagnosed, it begins a journey for the parents, a journey to acceptance and love. I fought so hard for so long against the reality that something was truly different about my girl. I missed the ausome blessing that was right in front of me for too long, but through my "road to Marion" encounter, my eyes were opened, and I began to see that God was using my little girl in amazing ways. I was connecting with people I never would have had the chance to connect with without autism. Also the way God uses Luci to speak directly to my soul makes me feel like I am living with a direct pipeline to heaven.

It was during this time that God opened my eyes to the work that he had been doing in my heart. I had spoken at a conference and someone came up to me to chat about what I had shared. I talked with her a little more in-depth about Luci and our story. She said, "It's so amazing the peace that radiates from you when you talk about Luci." We continued to talk, but I have to be honest, after she said that, my mind was not on the conversation at all. My heart literally skipped a beat when she said that about peace. The Holy Spirit used her words to grip my soul. My eyes were opened to the transformation that God had done in my life. I had become at peace with our story by becoming secure in his ausome love. Looking back I realized that I had experienced God's love in profound ways. I had felt it to the depth of my soul when Luci did something new or God made a way for us, and I had seen it surrounding and enveloping my daughter living life with a disability.

When I look back over the last thirteen years with Luci, I know God's love is ausome, because it's been the joy in our journey, the strength through our trials, the hope in the diagnosis. In Romans 8:37-39 we learn that "In all these things we are more than winners! We owe it all to Christ, who has loved us. I am absolutely sure that not even death or life can separate us from God's love. Not even angels or demons, the present or the future, or any powers can separate us. Not even the highest places or the lowest, or anything else in all creation can separate us. Nothing at all can ever separate us from God's love. That's because of what Christ Jesus our Lord has done."

And that is my ausome love story!

chapter 2

Ausomely Created

by Terry and Karen Bishir

From Karen:

Genesis 1:1: In the beginning God created...

Genesis 1:31: And God saw everything that he had made, and, behold, it was very good.

God's creation *never* ceases to amaze me. I see his love for me in an amazing sunrise and sunset. The vastness of our universe is beyond my comprehension. The animal kingdom brings us such joy. The intricate construction of our bodies is more than humans can totally understand. We are his workmanship. ("For we are his workmanship, created in Christ Jesus unto good works, which God hath before ordained that we should walk in them." —Ephesians 2:10)

He has patterned each of us, all of mankind (past, present, and future), in a very one-of-a-kind design. With God, there are no mistakes, no "oops," no "damaged goods," and no surprises. Should we doubt his sovereignty? Should we doubt his wisdom? Yes, doubts trouble us in the wee hours of the morning. But *should* we doubt his goodness to us? He is the source of our peace. John 14:27 says, "Peace I leave with you, my peace I give unto you: not as the world giveth, give I unto you. Let not your heart be troubled, neither let it be afraid." Meditate on Psalm 31:7: "I will be glad and rejoice in thy mercy: for thou hast considered my trouble; thou hast known my soul in adversities." We are called upon to "be strong in the Lord, and in the power of his might" (Eph. 6:10).

Luci is our first-born grandchild. I remember the day of her birth so well. Her parents (our daughter and son-in-law), my husband, and I were about one hour away from home at a couples' retreat sponsored by our church. In the early morning hours our phone rang. Our daughter Beth calmly informed us that she was pretty sure her water had broken. She was thirty-six weeks along in her pregnancy. We quickly made our way to their room. We were operating at a much faster pace than they were! We suggested that we leave immediately to make the trip to our local hospital. Once there and hooked to monitors, it was determined that Luci's heart rate significantly dropped with even the slightest contraction. After observing this for a period of time, it was determined that Luci would be born via a Caesarean section. Even though nothing seemed to be "textbook" about this birth, a healthy baby girl was born on October 16, 2004.

By all indications, Luci was a typical infant and toddler, but as the weeks gave way to months, there were signs of atypical behavior and development. Luci's language progression was not on target. There were other indicators that were causing alarm and worry. Luci's parents struggled to make sense of what they were seeing in their precious little girl. What did this mean? To whom could they turn? The days were passing, one by one, and still there were no answers. The urgency was evident and the stress was very real. We were all crying out to God for answers and for wisdom.

A diagnosis was given, but, in many ways, this only created additional insecurities, turmoil, and questions. These were dark and difficult days. The future was unclear, though God's grace, love, mercy, and strength were new every morning. Slowly, as the months became years, some answers have materialized. Many lessons have been learned. Much of God's character and love has been made abundantly clear.

These thirteen years have taught us many lessons. God has used the circumstances of our lives to mold and shape all of us, including Luci. He has placed within our heart an undeniable love for this very special granddaughter. He made her uniquely to be placed within our family. The love that I have for her has given me a deeper appreciation, love, and understanding for all of God's children. I am able to appreciate the uniqueness of every individual and to realize that we are all designed by an amazing Creator. Revelation 4:11 reminds us that, "Thou are worthy, O Lord, to receive glory and honour and power: for thou hast created all things, and for thy pleasure they are and were created."

I cling to the truth of Romans 8:28 *and* 29. "And we know that all things work together for good to them that love God, to them who are the called according to his purpose. For whom he did foreknow, he also did predestinate to be conformed to the image of his Son, that he might be the firstborn among many brethren." Notice that in verse 29, the ultimate purpose for "all things" is that we are conformed to his image. The ultimate goal for our earthly existence is to become Christ-like. Have we not been taught patience, humility, love, joy, peace, gentleness, and goodness through various circumstances that were not our choosing? Has our faith not grown as we place our utter confidence in what God can do in and through us? Have we not experienced the amazing sweet presence of his Spirit comforting us and filling us with his wisdom and strength? In these highs and lows, we see first-hand what God's presence brings to our lives. Psalms 91:2: "I will say of the Lord, He is my refuge and my fortress: my God; in him will I trust."

Let us contemplate Romans 11:33-36: "O the depth of the riches both of the wisdom and knowledge of God! How unsearchable are his judgments, and his ways past finding out! For who hath known the mind of the Lord? Or who hath been his counselor? Or who hath first given to him, and it shall be recompensed unto him again? For of him, and through him, and to him, are all things: to whom be glory for ever. Amen." Our focus must be one with eternity in view. Both good and bad can pull our focus from eternity. These verses in Romans challenge us to cherish the riches of his wisdom and his knowledge. His judgments and choices are beyond our understanding. It is so freeing to place *all* of our life at his feet and to live in total surrender to his plan and path for our life. For those of you reading this book, you, most likely, have a "Luci" in your life. My prayer is that you have already understood the immensity of his provisions for your life. His plan is perfect. When I accept that, my love for Christ grows exponentially. My love for others increases in ways that I am unable to truly understand. When I look at Luci, I see a beautiful granddaughter who is a direct gift from our loving Creator. Isaiah 43:7 says, "Even every one that is called by my name: for I have created him for my glory, I have formed him; yea, I have made him."

Yes, "In the beginning, God created..." God has created each and every one of us. But, oh, the beauty, strength, and confidence we gain from "and God saw everything that He had made, and, behold, it was very good." See the good. God's creation is good. I see it in words spoken for the first time. I see it when kisses are placed on the end of delicate fingertips and then placed on my cheek or shoulder. I see it in the unabashed excitement when spending uninterrupted afternoons in a pool where water can be poured out of the container over and over. I see it when the request of "Papaw, find me" is spoken during a ten-minute car ride from home to Kid's Praise at church. (Where does one hide in a car?) I see it when a request to go to heaven is as ordinary as a request to go to the park. I see it when letters on a page are transformed into words that are read for the very first time. I see it when an outing is actually enjoyable for all involved. I see it in the love that is displayed for siblings, family, pets, and special friends. I see it in tight hugs and beautiful smiles. I see it in the repeated requests to sing, "Jesus' Love is Bubbling Over." I see it in answered prayers for wisdom, transformed attitudes, friends, learning environments, and understanding. All of these answers to prayer are individual stories that could be told. Yes, "God saw everything that He had created, and, behold, it was very good." We, too, should marvel at his creation and proclaim, "It is very good."

From Terry:

By the time little Luci (our first grandchild) came into our family, I already had been in full-time ministry for over thirty years. As a pastor/teacher, my studies of the scripture had already brought me to a deep conviction concerning the sovereignty of God. God was in control. Circumstances in our lives didn't just happen without our Lord allowing them, and in reality, orchestrating them just the way he wanted things to be, both for his glory and our good. At first Luci seemed perfect and, of course, from this papaw's perspective, she was more than perfection. As time passed, concerns began to infiltrate our daily prayers. In time the reality became clear—our little Luci was more unique than most others. Even after the proper diagnosis, it took some time (really haven't gotten there yet) for me to use the proper title for her disability. *Wow,* I still struggle using that word disability. But as a Bible-believing Christian, I trusted that God in his sovereign love had not made a mistake, and that he had a holy purpose in this for Luci and each of us who were touched by this difficult opportunity.

John 9:1-3 teaches the true story of a blind man. When Jesus and his disciples passed by this man, his disciples asked Jesus, "Who did sin, this man, or his parents?" They were looking at this disability as a result of someone's sin. There is no doubt that, because we live in a sin-cursed world, all disability is a result of sin in a general sense and, on occasion, because of specific personal sin. Yet our great sovereign Lord can and will use disability for his glory and our good. Answering his disciples, Jesus explains that "neither this man sinned, nor his parents: but that the works of God should be made manifest in him." Jesus then proceeds to anoint this man's eyes with mud, and then commands him to go wash in the Pool of Siloam. The man obeys and immediately sees. There is so much in this passage, but the point Jesus makes clear is that the reason for this blindness was for God to display his power and great purposes in and through this man's disability.

Luci's life has not been easy for her or her family. Like the blind man, it has on occasion been difficult and expensive. Expensive in terms of time, treasure, emotions, and relations, but at the same time it has been filled with eternal dividends that only come through God as he chooses to manifest his glory and goodness through our disablements. Each new day I am made aware that Luci's divinely unique design has been one of God's great gifts to my life. I suspect that only eternity will reveal how many lives will be better because God is using her to teach and train us in his eternal ways, valuable ways, loving ways, and, above all else, Christ-like ways.

The Lord has used Luci Goosy (my affectionate nickname for her) in my life over these last thirteen years to help me be a better pastor, friend, husband, father, grandfather, and, I hope, a better child of God. There are so many ways that her life and particularly her uniqueness have impacted me for the better. Without the Lord sovereignly sending her to us, just the way she is, I would still be blind in so many areas. But because our Lord is working in her and for her, he is also working through her. It is as if he has chosen to give me sight in areas I would never have seen clearly without sight-giving lessons from her life.

I am certain that I am not the only one who has learned so much from Luci's daily life. There are events that are so sweet and, at other times, not so sweet. She has taught me to be more patient, especially with other families with children. I have learned to not pass judgment upon a child's behavior before I have all the facts and a full understanding. I have been taught to be more tenacious in my own disabilities; after all, no person alive is without disabilities of some sort. She reminds me to "not judge a book by its cover," but, instead, to look deep within a person. She has taught me to laugh more and I don't think anyone has made me smile more over the last few years than Luci. She teaches me the importance of being like Christ, as he protects the innocent, and loves unconditionally.

I am encouraged to be gentle with others as they struggle to learn and cope with life. I understand more fully the importance of remaining calm and in control of my emotions when others have "meltdowns" of any sort. I am learning that restraint often only causes reaction and rebellion. It is vital to find the balance between restraint and freedom as we relate with people of all ages. Childlike faith is what I desperately need. Luci's faith is amazing; tears flow when she suddenly begins to talk out loud to Jesus. Her connection with Jesus inspires me to stay in tune with my Lord on a twenty-four hour basis. To hear her pray leads me to trust in the Lord with all my heart. Her willingness to participate in activities and service opportunities at church and school encourages me to try new things that may be uncomfortable for me. When the Lord says, "walk into the water," I need to do just that. Her desire to forgive and not seek vengeance has moved me to seek the higher road as well. I see the great benefit of slowing down with life in general as I alter the pace of instructions, reading, and speaking when communicating with Luci. I am beginning to realize that people are listening even when it seems that they have tuned you out (Oh how this has helped me as I preach to my congregation!). Watching other children and adults accept and reach out in friendship to Luci has reinforced within me the importance of being a friend to everyone. Numerous lessons have been taught to me by a little girl who doesn't even know that she has become one of my greatest teachers of a lifetime.

Our Lord is so gracious to give us increased assets, which at first seem only liabilities. God has given the miracle of sight to me through this divinely created grandchild. So many things I have learned as I have gained insight through what could have been disabling. But because of faith in God's truth, deliverance has actually been the welcome outcome. Thank you, Lord, that your ways are not our ways and that your ways are better. Your plans and purposes are worth the difficulty and darkness that precede your deliverance and delight. (Today's darkness included an overflowing toilet on the second floor dripping through the ceiling of the first floor. Thanks, Luci for another lesson.) I am sure there will be more darkness in the days ahead, but I thank God for rays of divine light along the path. Staying focused on causes and not reasons will brighten one's day. In eternity it will be worth it all!

• • •

AUSOME THOUGHTS

Isn't it comforting to know that God has a plan?! His plans are not like our earthly plans. When God writes out our story in heaven, his plans are sovereign, infinite, and perfect. He created each of us with a specific purpose and plan in mind. When the unexpected happens in our life and we feel overwhelmed by handling life with a disability, our God is not perplexed. "Trust in the Lord with all your heart. Do not depend on your own understanding. In all your ways obey him. Then he will make your paths smooth and straight" (Prov. 3:5-6). By placing our trust in the goodness of his creation, we can have peace knowing that our life might be "plan b" to us, but it's exactly what God had planned all along. We are right where he planned for us to be and he is telling a beautiful story through the ausome blessing he created for his glory and our good.

—Beth

chapter 3

Ausome Opportunities

by Ryan Frank

G OOD THINGS COME TO THOSE who wait." I'm sure if you are anything like me, you have heard this cliché a million times. You wait for the perfect spouse, the perfect job, the perfect home, that dream car... and on and on we could go.

This saying has never been more real in our lives than with a young lady named Luci Frank.

I should rewind and introduce myself. Hi, I am Ryan. My amazing wife, Beth, is the author of this book. She's an amazing Christ-follower, student of the scripture, entrepreneur, and ministry partner, and is most amazing as a mom. We have three little girls who are our most important disciples. They are Lily, Londyn, and Luci.

Good things come to those who wait. Well, as Beth explained in Chapter 2, we waited for Luci. Infertility became a part of our lives early in our marriage. After several years of pain, waiting, and trusting, God gave us our firstborn daughter, Luci. It was worth the wait.

As Beth shared previously, God has allowed the Frank family to be ausomely blessed. Luci has autism. It hasn't been easy, but God has brought us to the point where we can say, "It is good."

Luci has brought lots of good things into our lives.

She makes us laugh. Laughing is good. It doesn't take much to make Luci giggle and in no time that giggle can turn into the loudest laugh you have ever heard.

She keeps us humble. Humility is good—especially with our personalities. Beth and I aren't really afraid of anything. We think we can do whatever we put our mind to and we can control any situation. That's absolutely not true, as we have learned with Luci.

She loves people. In a world full of evil and hate, love is good. Once Luci meets you, you are her friend. If you give her any attention at all, she is your best friend.

I could go on and on. Good things come to those who wait. We waited for Luci and we received something good. Even with the challenges that come with having a disability, Luci brings so much good into our family, church, and community. She makes us laugh, she keeps us humble, she loves people unconditionally, and so much more.

There's one other good thing that I want to mention. In fact, I'll probably spend a majority of this chapter talking about it. It's the *open doors* that have come by having an ausomely blessed child living under our roof.

God told a church once, "I know what you've been doing. Look! I have put in front of you an open door that no one can shut. You have only a little strength, but you have obeyed my word and have not denied my name" (Rev. 3:8, ISV). Pay attention to the phrase, "I have put in front of you an open door."

I'm going to let the pastor in me show here for a few minutes. I want to teach you about this verse and unpack it for you.

So much of our family's testimony can be found in this simple verse. I hope and pray it encourages you.

I love the Book of Revelation. It's the last book of the Bible, and some people are scared by it. Some people don't understand it. Others are fascinated by it.

I first fell in love with this book back in seminary. (I won't tell you how long ago that was!) I took a three-credit hour course just on this book. It was during this class that I really began to understand it with the Holy Spirit's help. It was one of the only college or seminary classes that I remember sitting on the edge of my seat in and taking notes in my Bible profusely.

If you have never studied the Book of Revelation, I encourage you to do it. It's the only book of the Bible that promises a special blessing to those who read it and do what it says. "The one who reads this is blessed, and those who hear the words of this prophecy and keep what is written in it are blessed" (Rev. 1:3, HCSB). If you have never studied Revelation, don't wait. Get your Bible open, get a good study guide, and ask the Holy Spirit to teach you.

When you get to Revelation 3, Jesus writes a letter to a church in the city of Philadelphia. The city of Philadelphia is a prosperous little Turkish town. It is located in a very beautiful valley that is inland a great distance, about 125-150 miles from the coast. The valley is a very wide one that runs north and south. The city was built on four or five hills in a picturesque setting.

The city didn't get its name (as many people think) from the Bible. Actually, the city got its name because of the love that Attalus II had for his brother Eumenes, who was king of Pergamum. Attalus had a great love and loyalty for his brother, and because of that it is called, "the city of brotherly love."

Enough history, let's get to the words that Jesus spoke to the church that was in that city. God said this, "I know what you've been doing. Look! I have put in front of you an open door that no one can shut. You have only a little strength, but you have obeyed my word and have not denied my name" (Rev. 3:8, ISV).

In this verse, the Lord praises and encourages the Philadelphian church for five things. I believe these words of Jesus can encourage you as well. Let's look at them.

First, Jesus says, "I know what you've been doing."

Did you know that the Lord didn't just know what *they* had been doing, but he knows what *you* have been doing? In fact, he is extremely interested in what is happening in your life.

It is often lonely when you have a child with special needs in your home. You don't feel like anyone can relate to your experiences. You don't feel support during times when you need it the most. You love when it's not easy. You give when you have no energy. You give yourself away when you are exhausted.

Know this, friend. God knows what you've been doing.

Listen to the precious words of the Scriptures:

Know that the LORD has set apart his faithful servant for himself; the LORD hears when I call to him. (Psa. 4:3, NIV)

In my distress I cried to the LORD; to my God I cried for help. From his Temple he heard my voice; my cry reached his ears. (Psa. 18:6, ISV)

The righteous cry out, and the LORD hears them; he delivers them from all their troubles. (Psa. 34:17, NIV)

The LORD is far from the wicked, but he hears the prayer of the righteous. (Prov. 15:29, NIV)

Those are beautiful words, but they are more than just beautiful. They are the truth! God hears you! He pays attention to your griefs and your loneliness and your heartaches. God pays attention and knows the problem before you are even sure of it yourself.

Second, Jesus says, "Look! I have put in front of you an open door that no one can shut."

What door had God opened to this church in Philadelphia? I'm not sure. It could have been a door to experience the joy and presence of the Lord like never before. Perhaps it was a supernatural knowledge of the scriptures. It could have been a huge ministry opportunity that opened. I like to believe it was just that—a big ministry opportunity of some sort.

Here's the point: God loves to open doors.

Did you know that God may be opening a door for you to do something big and hugely significant right now? It might come through your ausomely blessed kiddo. You might even miss it if you aren't looking. (Notice Jesus tells them to "look!")

Look around. What door is God opening? When he opens a door for you, he intends for you to peek inside. And that's not all ... he wants for you to walk inside, to investigate, to embrace and go full throttle with what he has given you.

Beth and I have seen so many doors open because of our Luci. We have been able to encourage people in our own community. We've helped parents and church leaders literally all over the world (which is so incredibly humbling). We have been able to partner with amazing ministries like Nathaniel Hope, Champions Club, and others who are trying to resource the home and church. Beth has been able to help people with this book and the resources available at AusomelyBlessed.com.

What door has God opened for you? Maybe it's a friendship with another parent. Maybe God is calling you to start a ministry in your community or church. Maybe God wants you to be a voice for those who can't speak up for themselves.

Here's the cool part. It's found at the end of the verse. God said, "I have set before you an open door, *which no one is able to shut.*" When God opens a door, guess what? It's not going to shut. Others may try to shut it. You might even try to shut it! But God won't let that door shut until you embrace it and see it come to life.

Let's keep moving. Look at the encouragement God gave next to this church.

Third, Jesus says, "You have only a little strength."

The word "strength" comes from the Greek word *dunamin*. *Dunamin* is where we get our English word *dynamite*.

Jesus said, "You have only a *little* strength."

While it can be a blessing to have a child with an intellectual or developmental disability, it can also be exhausting. You might feel like you have little power. Your strength is gone. You are exhausted. Guess what? God is very aware. He knew that this Philadelphian church lacked strength, and he knows when you do too.

I am tired. As Dr. James Dobson says, parenting isn't for cowards. It's tough work. But parenting a child with special needs takes things to a whole new level of fatigue. The good news? God knows "you have only a little strength."

I feel alone. It can feel lonely parenting a special needs child. While everyone else is bragging about how many words a minute their child can read, you are happy just to get yours to sit down for a few minutes to be read to. The good news? God knows "you have only a little strength."

I'm scared. What if I am not doing enough? Is there a new medication or therapy that I don't know about? How are other kids treating my child at school? What does the future hold? Fear is a daily reality for special needs parents. The good news? God knows "you have only a little strength."

I just want to talk to my child. Some of you will relate to this. Beth and I have often wondered what it would be like to have a "typical" conversation with Luci. What if she didn't have these special needs? What would she want to talk about? Where would she want to go? What would she want to say? Those questions cut deep in only a way that you can understand if you have experienced it. The good news? God knows "you have only a little strength."

The Apostle Paul once said this, "Each time he (God) said, 'My grace is all you need. My power works best in weakness.' So now I am glad to boast about my weaknesses, so that the power of Christ can work through me" (2 Cor. 12:9, NLT).

In a culture that promotes strength and independence, it may seem strange that weakness should be desired. Paul had asked the Lord to take away a "thorn of the flesh" that he was struggling with. However, this verse gives the Lord's response, as he tells Paul that God's power is made perfect in our human weakness.

In God's economy, his strength can shine through us more when we are weak. Here's why. When you are weak, you recognize your need for help. You acknowledge that you need something (or someone) bigger and stronger than you.

The very next words out of Paul's mouth were these, "For the sake of Christ, then, I am content with weaknesses, insults, hardships, persecutions, and calamities. For when I am weak, then I am strong" (2 Cor. 12:10, NLT).

"When I am weak, then I am strong." Let those words sink in. If you feel like you have little power today, be encouraged.

Fourth, Jesus says, "you have obeyed my word."

Back to the Book of Revelation, Jesus doesn't just write to the church at Philadelphia. He writes a letter to seven different churches in Asia. In every letter (with the exception of two) he has condemning words. The two churches our Lord gave no word of condemnation was Smyrna and this church, Philadelphia. Why? Because they had obeyed the Word of God.

God wrote a book. It's called the Holy Bible—the Word of God.

The Bible is comprised of sixty-six books written over a period of about 1,500 years by over forty authors from all walks of life, with different kinds of personalities, and in all sorts of situations. It was written in three languages on three continents, and it covers hundreds of controversial subjects. Yet, it fits together into one cohesive story with an appropriate beginning, a logical ending, a central character, and a consistent theme. How is this possible? Its author was God.

The Scripture says in 2 Peter 1:20-21, "Above all, you must understand that no prophecy of Scripture came about by the prophet's own interpretation of things. For prophecy never had its origin in the human will, but prophets, though human, spoke from God as they were carried along by the Holy Spirit."

The Holy Spirit revealed to the prophets the messages of the Bible. The writers of the Bible didn't write whatever they chose to write about, but only as they were moved, or controlled, by the Spirit of God. The Bible is a book written by God himself.

And get this: He wrote it with you in mind!

Too often we approach the Bible as a textbook—something thick, heavy, and dreaded. My prayer for you is that you would not view the Bible as a textbook, but as a love letter. A love letter is something you cherish and want to read over and over again.

Jesus encouraged the church at Philadelphia because they had obeyed his Word.

Sometimes it's not easy to do what God tells you to do. We must choose to obey God in faith. Every time we trust God's wisdom and do whatever he says to do, even when we don't understand it, we grow closer to God.

Remember this, though: we obey God because we love him and trust that he knows what is best for us, not out of fear or duty or compulsion. We want to follow Christ out of gratitude for all he has done for us, and the closer we follow Jesus, the deeper our relationship with him becomes.

When you obey what God tells you in his Word, it will release his power in your life. What are you afraid of right now? Whatever it is, it doesn't stand a chance when you do whatever

God tells you to do. There is no reason to be afraid. The Lord is on your side. Keep obeying his Word.

Fifth and finally, Jesus said, "you have not denied my name."

There is a great song that Jesus Culture sings called, "Break Every Chain." It pretty much repeats these words:

There is power in the name of Jesus
There is power in the name of Jesus
There is power in the name of Jesus
To break every chain
To break every chain
To break every chain

When life gets tough, when ministry gets tough, remember these words: There is power in the name of Jesus ... to break every chain!

The church at Philadelphia held tight to the name of Jesus.

In The Message Bible, Revelation 3:8 reads this way, "I see what you've done. Now see what I've done. I've opened a door before you that no one can slam shut. You don't have much strength, I know that; you used what you had to keep my Word. You didn't deny me when times were rough."

I love that. You didn't deny me when times were rough. Don't let go of the name of Jesus when times are rough. He has no plans of letting go of you.

Paul once said this, "We are hard pressed on every side, but not crushed; perplexed, but not in despair; persecuted, but not abandoned; struck down, but not destroyed" (2 Cor. 4:8-9, NIV).

No one wants to have their heart crushed. But being wounded in deep places happens. Life doesn't always seem fair. Sometimes it just seems to be a part of the rhythm of life.

And when these hard times come, we feel it all so very deeply. It impacts every part of our lives and it hurts. It's not normally during these times that we snap pictures and post them to Instagram and Facebook, right? Yet, we know Jesus is with us.

Here are six scriptures to remind you that you can trust Jesus to be with you in difficult times.

So do not fear, for I am with you; do not be dismayed, for I am your God. I will strengthen you and help you; I will uphold you with my righteous right hand. (Isa. 41:10, NIV)

The Lord is a refuge for the oppressed, a stronghold in times of trouble. Those who know your name trust in you, for you, Lord, have never forsaken those who seek you. (Psalm 9:9-10, NIV)

The LORD is good to everyone. He showers compassion on all his creation. (Psa. 145:9, NLT)

I have told you these things so that in Me you may have peace. You will have suffering in this world. Be courageous! I have conquered the world. (John 16:33, HCSB)

Don't worry about anything; instead, pray about everything. Tell God what you need, and thank him for all he has done. Then you will experience God's peace, which exceeds anything we can understand. His peace will guard your hearts and minds as you live in Christ Jesus. (Phil. 4:6-7, NLT)

For I can do everything through Christ, who gives me strength. (Phil. 4:13, NLT)

I hope that these words encourage you today. Ausome opportunities await you in your journey. Keep your eyes focused on the Lord and remember his words, "I know what you've been doing. Look! I have put in front of you an open door that no one can shut. You have only a little strength, but you have obeyed my word and have not denied my name."

• • •

AUSOME THOUGHTS

Life can seem so complex, but I love that life with Jesus is simplified. Simply trust him, simply obey him, and he gives us the grace and strength to do both of those things. As we live daily trusting and obeying, he takes us by the hand and he leads us on the most amazing God-adventures ever. How grateful I am that it's his strength I can rely on, when I have moments that don't feel like opportunities at all; moments that make me doubt the plan, moments when I just want an opportunity for normal—whatever that is. When we journey with Jesus, opportunity abounds in every ausome blessing, but it's up to us to seize the opportunities he brings our way for his glory and our good!

—Beth

chapter 4

Ausome Influence

by Craig Johnson

I HAD NO IDEA WHAT they were going through." "I just didn't know." These are the statements I hear over and over again when advocating for special needs from pastors, organizations, people, humanitarian groups, and the list goes on. How is it that special needs has been around forever and yet the challenges are still a mystery to most of society?

I'm sure there are many reasons that one could debate are the causes behind the lack of awareness. If it's not the hot topic at that time in society, it is easy to get overlooked. If families are so busy taking care of their child 24/7, shut in at their house, it's easy to be forgotten. When it's so challenging and it becomes an "event" just to go out from our house into the community, it can be so exhausting and difficult. Some have it much harder than others. My heart many times aches for them.

Yet, the flipside is that when we stay shut in because it's too exhausting and we're not out in the community, it's easy for someone to say, "I had no idea." I understand those cases where you are dealing with serious medical challenges that do not allow you to do what you would like for the sake of a special needs person's health. My heart is not to say who has it harder or who has it easier, that this is what they should do. I guess what I am saying is, how can we bridge the gap that brings more awareness where more people can understand and more people can connect in a positive way?

One thing that I've tried not to do in the journey with our son is let fear and obstacles stop us from living life and sharing about our son's amazing gifts and challenges. But it hasn't always been easy. One day all of the kids were playing out in the front of our street like neighborhood kids do. We had always been protective of Connor and I have to admit a little afraid of how others might treat him with his challenges. But that day Connor looked out the window and before I knew it, he was outside running and jumping around the other kids yelling, "Yahoo!" My first inclination was to go out and bring him in so they wouldn't stare at him like any child would who didn't understand. But I waited. It was the Spirit of God prompting me not to intervene. Under my breath I'm praying, "Please let them go on playing or please let one of the kids be nice to him." It was wishful thinking because the next thing I knew every ball dropped to the ground, everyone stopped what they were doing, and everyone with a weird look on their faces just stared. My heart sunk. Immediately I wanted to go out and bring Connor in so he could be safe and protected. But then I heard God speak to me, "Who are you protecting, Connor or your feelings?" Wow! God knows how to ask the questions that we don't always want to hear.

So instead of walking out there to take my son in, I walked out there, put my arm around my son, and asked the kids if they knew what autism was. Everyone shook their heads no. So I began to explain to them about Connor and why he reacts differently and what makes him so unique. Then something beautiful happened. One of the more popular girls on the block asked if she could play with Connor. Surprised, I said sure. And for the next thirty minutes they played in Connor's clubhouse and she observed Connor and interacted with him. The next week I came home from work and I heard in the backyard Connor counting down, "5-4-3-2-1- blast off!" And there was Connor holding hands with three girls on one side and three girls on the other side jumping into the pool. Every boy in the neighborhood would have probably liked to be Connor at that point. Ha! He was having a blast!

Now all the kids in our neighborhood understand what Connor has but don't look at him the same way they did before we came out of the house and shared his life with them. Sometimes people don't know because we're too protective or afraid to let them know. It's safer in protective areas like our house. But if we really want to see our kids grow and bring awareness, sometimes we have to take a chance and go outside.

When I moved from sunny Southern California to Seattle, Washington, it was a big change. When it rained in California, we would usually go inside. That's what you did. So the first six months while living in Seattle, because it was raining most of the time, we almost became shut-in's. We hardly ever went out to play or interact with people. It got depressing basically moving from one building to the next. Then one day I talked to a Seattle native and I said, "Don't you ever get depressed staying in because it's so cloudy and raining all the time?" He said, "We don't stay in. We golf in the rain, play in the rain, we do all sorts of things in the rain. It rains here 260+ days out of the year. If you don't get out in the rain, you don't live life fully."

Those of us who are special needs families can feel the same way. More days than not we can feel like it's always overcast, always raining (figuratively speaking). So instead of pushing through, we stay shut in most of the time. We hardly ever get out and interact with people. Maybe people don't know about us because people rarely see us. It's not until we decide to go out even in the rain (challenges) that we can live life to the fullest. My son would have never made that connection with those boys and girls if we would have kept him "protected" in the house.

Maybe the more out and about people see us, the more conversations and awareness can take place so that one day instead of hearing people say, "I had no idea," they will say, "I know him!"

I don't think in the beginning when someone looks at a child with special needs, the first thought that comes to mind is "greatness." I mean how can something that on the outside some people would assume deficient have the best chance for greatness? This is how the finite human mind works. If something doesn't appear to have promise, how can it be promising? If it doesn't appear to be beautiful, how can it be beautiful? I'm glad God doesn't look at things the way some people do. How many miracles would we have missed if God didn't help us see the possibility? One of the greatest gifts God gives to us is helping us understand that potential is not realized because someone started out with all the perfect ingredients. Potential is realized when someone sees the flower in the seed. No one is ever born great; they develop greatness. Somebody saw the potential of the destiny before the destiny was realized. They had to look deeper than the circumstance. They had to live in the vision and not the circumstance.

In the Old Testament if the people of Israel were to compare the strapping stoic King Saul to scrawny no-'count David from the outside, it wouldn't have even been a contest. Saul would win in a landslide. He would have been the people's pick to be king. No one would have seen the possibility of David being king. Even David's own father showed the prophet Samuel every one of his other sons before he presented David. Why? Because David didn't look like a king from the outside. Yet, I have found who we think should be king may not be who God thinks should be king. The enemy will try to cover up greatness with our children. The enemy will put up weeds to choke the seed of greatness in them. He wants to blind us from what could be so we will accept what we have. When we reflect on God's view of people and we see the world from his perspective, we are removing the weeds that choke out what's possible. When our hearts are ready, we are able to see the destiny seeds in others.

Oliver Wendell Holmes once said, "What lies behind us and what lies ahead of us are tiny matters compared to what lives within us." Man looks on the outside but God looks deep within and looks at the heart. Where it really becomes powerful is when he gets us to believe there is something great inside someone else even when no one else sees it. Who would have ever seen greatness in Helen Keller from the outside? She was blind, deaf, and mute—three strikes against greatness. Her destiny would seem to be just to survive. Especially in the era she lived in, when they had far fewer tools and medical know-how to develop multiple special needs. Yet her teacher saw a destiny seed of greatness that God had planted. She saw an amazing flower that could blossom in the midst of what others would call barren seed. She called forth greatness when others would have gotten frustrated and given up. Helen Keller became a great American hero in spite of her challenges because someone watered what God had already sown. The greatest legacy is not what we leave for people; it's what we leave in people.

Sometimes you cannot just hope for greatness; you have to call it forth. With our kids we may have to speak it over them every day and call forth the greatness of the destiny seed God has planted inside of them. Speaking everyday over them: my child is talented, my child is creative, my child is healed, my child is a masterpiece, my child will do great things. God is not moved by our circumstance. He is moved by our faith. He understands, he is compassionate, he loves us, but what he is really moved by is our belief that he can do anything. When it looks impossible, do we still believe?

From the time our son Connor was one and saying his first word to almost two years old, he was a chatterbox. This was somewhat normal to us. Our other two children Cory and Courtney, who are ten and twelve years older than Connor, were the same way. They talked incessantly. We thought every child did this. My son Cory at a very young age would watch a video called *Super Book* about David and Goliath. He would walk around with a plastic sword and cloth sling and proclaim as he swung his sling, "I will slay you Gowiath (Goliath) in the name of the Loward (Lord) for him is on my side!" The imaginary stone would be thrown and he would run over and knock down a toy transformer. Then he'd pull his sword out, and with a mighty swing cut off the transformer's head, which we had to tape back on over and over. Then, and as he held the transformer's head in his hand, he would proclaim, "God has dewivered this Philwistine into my hand!" I don't know how Biblically correct it was but it was hilarious watching him do this. This is normal right? Every kid does this.

When Connor was two, he would say "I love you" without hesitation. Then all of a sudden he said nothing. Where he would play with other kids, all of a sudden he would sit in a corner and only play by himself. What at one time seemed ordinary now would become a miracle. Because for the next three years, we would barely hear our son put two words together.

It's interesting what we take for granted in life because it happens so naturally or is so abundant to us.

I remember the first hurricane I ever experienced after coming to Houston. When the 100 mph winds and rain finally stopped, there was no electricity and no running water for multiple days. What seemed so ordinary a few days ago became in an instant so scarce.

The truth is that life is a miracle. There are miracles happening around us every day. The very things we get used to because they seem effortless, if taken away, would become a miracle.

No one understands that more than a special needs parent. When you were preparing with joy and excitement to have your new baby, you must have dreamed about all the things they were going to do just like any other child. But, it didn't turn out that way. God had a scarier, bigger plan. You thought your child would do ordinary things like others, but God was going to show you that you will see miracles no one else can see.

For instance, anyone can get a drink of clean water in America. Seems ordinary right? Yet it would be a *not so ordinary miracle* for a child in Africa, where the only water they have access to is dirty and diseased. Having a healthy child would seem pretty ordinary for most parents, right? Yet, to my friend and fellow blogger Barb Dittrich, who has seen her children in and out of hospitals for years, this would be an amazing miracle. A little girl having a conversation with her mommy seems fairly ordinary for many parents, don't you think? But, for my wife Sam and I to hear one sentence from our son after years of silence would be beyond a miracle.

For three years we barely heard him speak. He would point to things he needed. Because he couldn't speak, he would get frustrated and act out. Sometimes it would be terrible fits; other times it would be biting or scratching his arms. I remember one day driving to work, I asked God why. I wasn't asking God why I had my son; I was asking God why is my son not able to speak? Why does he have to struggle so much in frustration?

I'll never forget what God spoke to me in my spirit. God said, "Your child is not a burden; your child is a gift." I said, "I know what you mean, God, he's our son, we love him, of course he's a gift, but do you see how much he's struggling?" God said it again, "Your child is not a burden; your child is a gift. You are looking at the struggle and not seeing how I can use your test and make it a testimony. I am going to use your son to reach millions of people." I said, "Are you kidding me, God? How is my son going to reach millions of people? Right now he can't even ask for a drink of water?" Then God said four words that he will always say to those who feel like they are in the desert. He said, "*Do you trust me?*" I gave God a very simple and vulnerable answer. I said, "You are all we've got in this situation. There is no cure for autism but you. *We trust you.*" God later said to me, "Thank me for the miracles I am already doing, every day, all around you, and watch me do the miracles yet to be seen. Your son is alive; that's a miracle. There are moms and dads who can't have children that would be so proud to have a son like Connor. Your son gives you a hug and a kiss when you ask; that's a miracle. Many children with autism don't do that. Thank me for the *not so ordinary miracles* and watch me surprise you with my goodness."

You think it's going to get easier after you hear God speak like that, right? It didn't. It got worse. After God speaks, many times, he is wanting to see if we will trust him and thank him. Praise precedes the victory. Psalm 50:14-15 says, "Make thankfulness your sacrifice to God, and keep the vows you made to the Most High. Then call on me when you are in trouble, and I will rescue you, and you will give me glory."

About three months later my wife, who was putting our son to bed, started yelling, "Craig, Craig get up here! Hurry!" So I ran upstairs, walked into my son's room and said, "What is the matter?" My wife Sam said, "I was putting Connor to bed, reading a book, praying with him, and as I went to turn off the light, all of a sudden he begin to speak. One word after another word, one sentence after another sentence." I said, "You have got to be kidding me? What ... what did he say?" She walked me over to his bed and said, "Connor, say it again, say it for daddy." He lifted up his head and in broken English all of a sudden began to speak, "This is my Bible, I am what it says I am, I have what it says I have, I can do what it says I can do. Tonight I will be taught the Word of God. I boldly confess, my mind is alert, my heart is receptive, I will never be the same. I am about to receive the incorruptible, indestructible, ever-living seed of the Word of God. I will never be the same, never, never, never, I will never be the same in Jesus' name. Amen." Those were the first sentences we had heard him speak since he had stopped speaking. To say we were overwhelmed would be an understatement. We were crying, hugging, jumping, and yelling. We called everyone we knew and videotaped Connor saying, "This Is My Bible..." and now millions of people have heard that testimony. It has been written about in five books; it was the inspiration to launch Champions Club developmental centers for special needs kids around the world.

God showed us something powerful through all of this. Try not to look at the burden—focus on the gift. Emily Colson's dad, Chuck Colson, wrote that when he had shared with close friends about his grandson being diagnosed with autism, a good friend sent him a note that read, in part, "With your grandson you have been given the greatest gift. Now, you will truly understand what it means to sacrificially love."

Celebrate what we do have, not what we don't have. We have so much to be grateful for and our kids have so much to give. An intellectual or developmental disability doesn't stop special needs kids from making an impact on the world around them. Even though lots of these kids face communication challenges, they are able to share God's love in powerful ways. God will use them if we allow them to be used to have awesome influence. Our job is to point these kids and families to their destiny and help them navigate how to get there.

• • •

AUSOME THOUGHTS

How exciting to think that with God a disability is actually the ability to influence! A diagnosis isn't a mandate to watch life from the sidelines, but a call to a destiny of greatness: "But I had a special reason for *making you king* (or giving you a disability, my emphasis). I decided to show you my power. I wanted my name to become known everywhere on earth" (Ex. 9:16). God has called every believer to a life of significance. Sometimes we don't want to be significant in the way that he has called us to be, but ausome influence is a calling and not a choice. Jesus, help us to step out into the destiny that you have called us to. May our ausome blessings influence the world greatly for you!

—Beth

chapter 5

We Love Luci

Stories of how God shows up miraculously in the everyday and has brought friends, healing, and peace through the community he has built around our ausome blessing, Luci.

I LOVE LUCI! I HAD the privilege of being Luci's school-teacher for three and a half years! She was a joy to work with! My most favorite thing about Luci was her laugh! She loves life and loves to laugh! I enjoyed laughing with Luci! I also loved that Luci had lots of friends. The kids in her three general education classes were so helpful and they enjoyed playing with Luci! So many great memories of Luci! She brightened my day when she would enter the room and yell at the top of her lungs, "Schwarze, you okay?" We had lots of fun on field trips, going bowling, riding horses, swimming, going to Conner Prairie, and going to the Pumpkin Patch. We've started a new school year and Luci has moved to a new school. I miss her a bunch but cherish the years I had with her in my classroom! I love Luci!

—Brenda Schwarze

I love Luci! She has half of the storage on my phone from all of the videos she makes! I was so proud of her during kids' camp! She did things that I thought she wouldn't even think about doing! I had so much fun spending a couple of days with her! My favorite memory with her is when she was sitting by me at the service at kids' camp. Sarah, our children's pastor, was hitting her husband, Mike, with a bat to show the helmet of salvation. Then Luci decided she wanted to hit him too. She stood up and walked up to the front and said, "My turn!" Mike said, "no!" (I don't know why) and she sat by me again and was mad/sad the rest of the service. Haha!

—Alyssa Carmichael

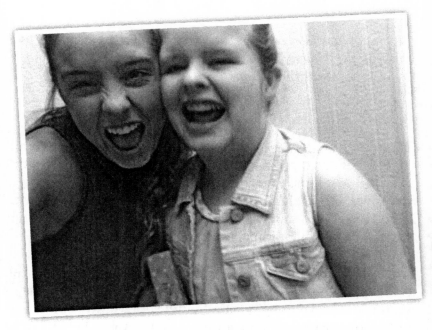

One of my favorite memories of Luci is of her being a part of our wedding. It is so precious to Matt and me that we were able to share that with her. Of course her laugh, sense of humor, and love for snacks always bring a smile to my face. I love how after we moved, she found where the snacks were very quickly and she also found prime echo spots. One being on the stairway to the basement, and another at the picnic table in the backyard. I love to hear her yell and then crack up when she hears herself echo back. I also cherish the special bond her and Ellie share. Ellie is up for anything Luci wants to do, when no one else is. That is ultimate trust right there, lol. (I wish I had a pic of the mini moto adventure!) We love Luci and are so very thankful for her!

—Megan Bishir

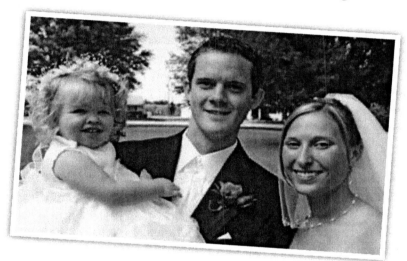

I remember Luci being in my Life Skills class at Sweetser during my first year of teaching a new class. Boy did Luci keep me on my toes! She is goofy, yet sweet. She sure loved to work for M&Ms! I probably should've bought stock in them that first year as I was constantly buying them! She also made sure we got our exercise, I imagine to help burn off the M&M calories, when she would decide to take off from the kindergarten classroom and through the halls of Sweetser! The couple of years that I taught her, it was a joy to praise her in each accomplishment she had: speaking, sitting still, following directions, and learning!

—Jillian Matteson

Luci wants to drive the bus! Maybe next Tuesday? I am blessed to be her bus driver! I love her telling me she loves me to the moon and back! I love that I have to invite her on the bus every morning and kick her off in the afternoon! I love that she pats the top of my head! I love that she loves to sing! We sing "Three Little Monkeys"! I love her hair! I love how excited she is with different people waiting on her after school. (I know the favorite but I will keep that to myself!) I love it when she tells me "We are *going* to Abby's today." I love the way she touches your hand or shoulder so tenderly. I love to hear her talk! I love to hear her laugh! I love it when she says, "I see my house, Miss Dana," and we are in Swayzee, several miles away! I love it when her grandpa puts her on the bus. Hair may not be combed just right, but she is happy! I love the way she loves chocolate chip cookies! I love the way God placed Luci in the perfect family! I love Luci!

—Dana Hueston

We've only known Luci and her family for a couple of years, but have had many times together where we have learned about Luci, and it seems like she always leaves us with a smile—and most of the time a giggle—on our faces. I remember the first time she and her family came over. She was organizing our shoes in the garage. Beth apologized over and over, but I told her, "Don't apologize! It's not bothering me at all. What else does she want to organize for me?!"

One summer, we had Luci and her family over to our house and the kids were all playing outside. We have a red wagon that my husband, Doug, had been pulling the kids around in. Luci got her ride in the wagon and every time Luci sees Doug now, she wants to come to our house to ride in the red wagon. We have promised her she could come anytime she wants for that red wagon ride. We find it funny that she remembers that and that it is the first thing she asks for every time! The simplicity of a wagon ride.

Luci was at the lake last summer. A friend and I stayed back and watched all the kids (and by all, I mean ten kids ages newborn and up—what were we thinking?!) while the rest of the adults went on a boat ride. Luci kept walking in the house and grabbing snacks, which I didn't mind, but I knew Ryan and Beth didn't want her doing that as she had continually asked them for snacks beforehand. I kept trying to sidetrack her away from the snack table, but she wasn't having it! So I remember walking out to my friend and saying, "She won't stop eating ... I don't know how to get her to stop eating!" Lol. Both of us tried to get her to stop, but all of our tactics weren't working well. So, if I remember correctly, she had a good share of snacks that day and when the boat returned and they asked how everyone did, our response was, "Oh they were great, no problem!" Haha!

What I love about Luci the most, though, is her love for the little things. How she finds joy in a red wagon, laughing, and even yelling. She helps us grow in our teaching and communication as we strive to serve her in the best way we can. She teaches us humility and strength. She is a true gift from God, who keeps all of us on our toes.

—Whitney Kingseed

When I think of Luci Frank, I can't help but smile. Being her aunt is one of life's greatest blessings. One of my favorite Luci moments happened last summer. She had just gotten back from church camp and we were having a cousin sleepover. She kept asking me to sing one of her camp songs, "Crank It Like a Chainsaw." I'm sure I said twenty times, "Crank it like a what?" After learning the lyrics we sang it every way I could think of, opera, country, and rap style, slowly, loudly, and quietly. She could hardly get it out, she was laughing so hard, followed by, "Again, Kristy, again!" Luci laughs and Luci "love taps" are some of my favorite things. She is persistent and has a genuine love for her people! I love that those who know her best know that if you fall or get hurt, she's going to find it hilarious, and it's okay! It's been an amazing thirteen years watching Luci grow into the special girl that she is and watching her parents fight for her along the way. Luci loves big and full and being loved by her is one of the best things in the world!

—Kristy Frank

One of my favorite Luci memories is from camp several years ago. I was Luci's camp counselor and watched over her at night. She did great the first night but the second night I remember having to text Ryan because Luci was laughing uncontrollably that night in the dark cabin. I still remember Ryan coming to pick her up. She kept telling me about giving her stuffed dog a bath or something along those lines. When I look back at the pictures from camp that year, it reminds me of the little Luci and how far she has come as I teach her now Sunday mornings!

— Elizabeth Bollhoefer

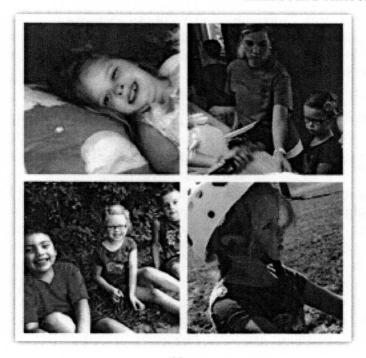

Luci was my introduction to "unclehood" and what a blast it's been. Anytime we're in a car, it's a *dance party*, literally. She gives the best high fives of anyone I know. She knows all my "snack spots" around the house and that's her first stop anytime she's over! One quick funny Luci story: One night years ago she was staying over and in the middle of the night I was having the weirdest dream that a cat was walking along the edge of the bed. (We did not own a cat.) I kept seeing this "cat" and realized all of a sudden I wasn't dreaming! Luckily I didn't swing at it or anything because it was just Luci standing beside the bed watching me sleep! Her hair was at just the right level that it looked like an animal! She's a special girl with a special place in my heart! I love Luci!

—Nick Frank

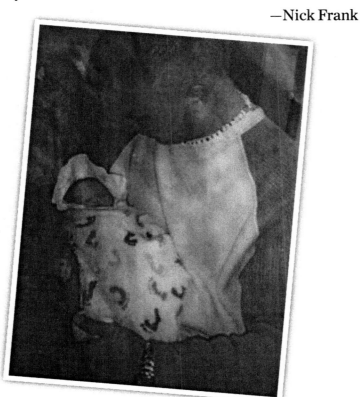

"Aunt Paula, find me!!!" I can hear Luci, my great-niece, saying those words from a few years ago. Such a fun way to think of the little girl, now growing into a teenager. One day after a family party I told Luci I would "find her" and pretended I couldn't see her—like hide and seek. When I "found" her she giggled and giggled. I think we played "find Luci" 20 times in that 15 minutes. So fun! Every time I saw Luci after that, whether at church or anywhere, she wanted me to find her.

One of the best memories of Luci is in Sunday School. I was privileged to be her Sunday School teacher for two years! Luci didn't communicate a lot then. What a wonder how far she has come! I love Luci and will never forget being her teacher. Now she is in my AWANA class, and she has gone from "Find me, Aunt Paula" to "Can I stay at your house?!" Now that is a memory I am ready to make! Being with Luci is a gift. She brings sparkle into my day everytime I see her!

—Paula Davis (Aunt Paula)

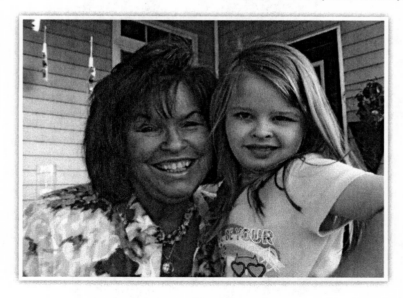

chapter 6

Ausome Innocence

by Emma Roudabush

*Do all things without grumbling or disputing; so that you
will prove yourselves to be blameless and innocent, children
of God above reproach in the midst of a crooked and perverse
generation, among whom you will appear lights in the world.
— Philippians 2:14-15*

I STARTED WORKING WITH CHILDREN with autism over
five years ago. My first week on the job I ended up at Med-
Check with an open bite wound on my arm. I considered
quitting that day. I thought, "What kind of job allows you to
get bitten?" I was not prepared for biting. Surely there were
other much more qualified, patient, stronger-skinned people
than me to "handle" children like this. My perspective and understanding of these children then was limited and distorted.
I wouldn't have described the biter as *innocent* at that time
but God continued to open my eyes, open doors, and lead me
to work in the autism field. I would like to share some of this

journey with you through stories of people in my life who have opened my eyes to the way God uses and works through innocence.

My church offers a program for adults with disabilities. Every year they have an overnight camp where a person with a disability is partnered with a volunteer without a disability. It's a fun camp with tons of activities and laughs but it often takes some serious persuading to get volunteers to sign up to spend a few days and a couple nights in this setting. It's always encouraging to see the new volunteers' perspectives shift.

My first year at camp I was partnered with Kelsey. Kelsey has Down syndrome and immediately considered me her best friend (she found a boyfriend at camp pretty quickly too). We wrapped up our first day of activities and gathered with the large group for worship. The worship songs began and Kelsey began shouting her praises to the Lord. There were many words she didn't know and her speech was inarticulate but when the main verses came around she sang as loudly as she could. Many turned and looked at Kelsey but she didn't seem to notice. She held her hands up and genuinely praised God. It was beautiful.

When it came time for devotion, Kelsey asked to hold my hand. I couldn't help but think, "Doesn't she see others looking at us? Doesn't she care what others think about her?" In reality, I think she's got more figured out than me. Wouldn't life be better spent if we all loved and worshiped so deeply, so freely, so innocently? Whether Kelsey knows it or not, she is fulfilling the greatest commandments. She's loving God and loving people. "Make a joyful noise unto the Lord, all the Earth; make a loud noise, and rejoice, and sing praise" (Psa. 98:4).

Innocence can be defined as harmless in intention. When I think of innocence in this sense, I think of the greeter at my local grocery. This particular greeter seems to be working every time I run to the grocery. He greets with a smile and always gives a compliment. Sometimes, you get two or three right when you walk in the door. My most recent trip to the grocery I was greeted with something like this, "Welcome! You look beautiful today. Are you related to Cinderella? You look just like her with your hair like that. I like your boots. Here's a cart." I didn't even get a chance to say hello before the cart was heading my way.

It should be noted that my hair looked nothing like Cinderella. Though, he *could* have been referring to her hair in her "servant cleaning house" days in which case may have been totally accurate. To be honest, some people walk in and laugh at him or think he's strange. He does have an arm that he holds by his side and his compliments and comments are often awkward or over the top, but he always seems to be able to put a smile on every face. His innocence is beautiful and completely harmless in intention—wrapped in pure kindness, pure joy. Some people just seem to radiate innocence like that. The best part is that we all have the opportunity to live like this through our faith because God defines innocence as freedom from sin. Some of us have a harder time grasping this innocence and living as free sons and daughters of God.

Individuals with autism have a different view of the world, which brings with it a set of diverse struggles and challenges. In fact, individuals with autism have brains that actually look and function differently. Their brains tend to focus on one task at a time, rather than multitasking. Their brains tend to focus on facts and rules; struggle with complex tasks; enjoy routines, schedules, and repetitive tasks; and have difficulty in social settings.[1] Knowing this about their brain function enables others to engage in a way that promotes further understanding and success.

---

1. Buron, Kari Dunn. et al. *Learners on the autism spectrum: preparing highly qualified educators.* Shawnee Mission, KS, AAPC, 2008.

For example, in general, it's better to communicate with a few direct words, provide assistance or prompts in unstructured social situations, and to acknowledge that something which may appear simple or easy to you or me may be challenging and need to be taught in multiple ways on numerous occasions in order to be learned by someone with autism. As a behavior consultant my job is to change or replace bad behavior. Studying behaviors is really quite interesting because as you study them, you learn that behaviors happen for a reason. When I look to change a behavior, the focus of my plan leans on the function of a behavior or why a particular behavior is happening. Once the root of the behavior is revealed, it becomes much simpler to address the behavior.

Oftentimes the behavior has little to do with malicious intent but is merely a communication error. To put it simply, the person with a disability does not know how to appropriately communicate when they want attention, need a break, or are frustrated. Bad behaviors are used to communicate when appropriate behaviors have not yet been acquired. Once we are able to understand the undesired behavior from the perspective of the child, we can and should teach alternative ways of achieving the same desire. Good behaviors and progress should then be rewarded. For me, this understanding resulted in a shift of thinking—a shift in the way I engaged with people in general. Bad behavior should not automatically be punished but new behaviors should be taught, reinforced, altered, and practiced.

It would be impossible for me to create a general description for children with autism. While children with disabilities can display many similarities, they are also exceedingly diverse. Some can quote entire movies, some are mute, some enjoy music, some can compute long numbers, some avoid eye contact, some enjoy holding hands, some are fascinated with narrow interests, some rock back and forth, some are aggressive, and some give too many kisses. Behaviors can be changed and nurtured and developed. I don't think God created all children to be alike or to fit in some sort of one-size-fits-all box, but God did create children to be loved and to engage. My goal is to ensure that these children are taught how to engage. But, this work can be scary. This work can be faith-testing.

My work with children with autism led me to meet Stewart. After working at my previously mentioned job for some time, I began to want to work with children with more challenging behaviors, and they gave me Stewart. He was a wild one. His mom would drop him off every morning looking exhausted. He was full of energy and pretty destructive. I was able to develop a relationship with Stewart's mom and I was given the insight of what it is like having a child with a disability. Stewart's mom confided in me her worries and her fears. It seems that oftentimes we let our fear control our actions. We are afraid because we do not understand the disability, we are afraid that we don't know how to help, and we are afraid to get involved and fail. To empathize with her struggles allowed me to be more willing. There were many times when I failed with Stewart, when I'm sure I did more harm than good. There were also times when we celebrated victories such as asking someone to play with him or getting a drink by himself. I'm no longer working with Stewart but I'm sure that he is still making progress toward a more meaningful life, a life of freedom because of others who don't let fear stand in their way.

After working with Stewart I met one of my best friends. She was blond hair, blue eyes, one of the best senses of humor, and autism. Our relationship didn't start out with jokes or going to the movies. As her behavior consultant I had a plan for improving her language, her compliance, and her independence. As it often goes, she changed my behavior too. In the beginning she would often run and hide from me; there were times I would have to pick her up and bring her back to the table. There were days when she would yell. There were days when I would cry on my way home because I didn't understand, I wasn't doing enough, and it felt like failure. Other times it felt like everything was right in the world and I could see so obviously God's purpose for her life. I didn't expect friendship. As we began to work together and I got to know Luci, I found that she had the type of humor that makes everyone smile. She is sweet and innocently ornery. There have been many times that I found myself leaving her house filled with joy. I looked forward to our times together because we would laugh and learn and love.

As time passes, I tend to value friendships more and more. I treasure friends who are honest, who laugh, who are nonjudgmental, and who embody innocence. Luci is exactly that kind of a friend. She improves my life and I work to improve hers. Proverbs 27:17 exemplifies this saying: "As iron sharpens iron, so a friend sharpens a friend." Sadly, people with disabilities don't often have meaningful friendships. Luci has shown me that this should not be the case. I think we can foster and embody what it means to encourage meaningful friendships by teaching children with and without disabilities how others think and communicate, to break down the barriers and promote acceptance of differences. This may look like awkward silence and weird role playing or scripted conversations at first, but I truly believe something beautiful can come from this. It's possible that friendships can best be taught by modeling this behavior as adults.

In considering my memories of working with people who have disabilities, I'm continually reminded of the innocent perspectives they embody and how this affects how they view the world. I'm so thankful that God maintains patience with me and allows each of these people to influence my life. Many people with disabilities don't see the world the way I do. While I spend too much of my time chasing money, acceptance, and peace, they often don't value money, don't care much what others think, and have a sense of freedom that I so often forget. How much time of my own life do I waste caring what others think about me when I could spend that time valuing people and the beauty of life instead? It's easy to see the behaviors that need to be changed or fixed without taking the time to appreciate the behaviors that are so beautiful.

I once heard a pastor say something that has persisted in my thoughts over the years. It was a moment in his sermon as he explained that the word "awesome" was too often used. The word means to stand in awe. Synonyms include overwhelming, breathtaking, splendid, humbling, and fearsome. You can describe the post of your Facebook-worthy food or the World Series home run as being "awesome" but in reality there are few things that are as awesome as experiencing the power and presence of God. When you experience the innocence and beauty that comes from genuinely loving people and seeing God's handiwork, then you have experienced something that is truly awesome: the night sky, laughter, the greeter at the grocery, tiny dimpled hands, right words that come just when you need them. It takes your breath away; it reminds you that God's got our worries, our messes, and our fears figured out and he is in control. Opportunities for awe are ever present and noticing them often just requires a shift in perspective. We stand in awe because our God is an awesome God.

As I am sitting here writing this now, I am holding my newborn baby girl and I can't help but be in awe of God. I'm in awe of her intricacies, the way her chest rises and falls, her fingers as she grabs mine, and her eyes as they flutter off to sleep. I'm in awe that God would allow me to be a mother to his creation. As children grow and life's demands muddle our spiritual focus, it is easy to forget how beautiful the miracle of life is—the innocence and pureness of life. It becomes ever more important to remember that God divinely created every person in this world. He's the one who created our unique gifts. It is assuring to know that even if someone may seem incomplete, they are created exactly how God designed them to be. Exodus 4:11 says this well: "The Lord said to him, 'who gave human beings their mouths? Who makes them deaf or mute? Who gives them sight or makes them blind? Is it not I, the Lord?" Breathe that truth in.

We all have the opportunity to be innocent because Jesus died and forgave our sins on the cross so that we may be harmless and pure. Let us take inspiration from those around us who model this innocence so well. I would challenge you today to take the time to see the world through a different perspective. To take the time to look past the behavior and into the heart of a person. To allow yourself to be vulnerable and willing. I'm challenging you because of how thankful I am that God has allowed me to see the world through innocent, ausome eyes.

• • •

AUSOME THOUGHTS

Living in a society that values "street smarts" sometimes makes it hard to appreciate the true gift of guilelessness. There is so much bad in our world today that is hard to handle and understand. Without even realizing it, I become a little wearier, a little heavier after watching the morning news. I believe it's a true blessing that individuals with an intellectual or developmental disability see the world more like God intended it to be, more like it was in the Garden of Eden. Holding a grudge, being devious, or manipulating a situation is not something that most of these kiddos ever struggle with. What is more beautiful in the body of Christ than innocent eyes, looking on the world around them with love and joy, innocent hands holding on to Jesus and trusting him completely in the good times and the bad? I say "nothing compares."

—Beth

chapter 7

Ausome Potential

by Doc Hunsley

WHAT DO YOU SEE WHEN you see an individual with special needs? Way too many people see an individual who is defined by a diagnosis, and that is just wrong! I see ausome potential! I see individuals who are fearfully and wonderfully made in the image of God! I see individuals with amazing abilities, who can do amazing things! I see some of my heroes! I see difference makers! I see Kingdom builders!

God has blessed my life the past thirteen years and has developed an undeniable passion in me for individuals and families with special needs. Initially, I was someone who first saw an individual with special needs as defined by their diagnosis. I was a pediatrician in a pediatric emergency room, where I cared for many children with special needs. I knew they had lots of love to give, but I didn't see much more beyond that.

Then God allowed me to become really sick from my patients and almost die; I was forced to go out on long-term disability. This happened around the time my second son, Mark

Andrew Hunsley, was born. Eight months later he had a seizure that lasted over four hours and around eighteen months of age he was diagnosed with Dravet syndrome, a rare genetic seizure disorder. By two, he received his second diagnosis of autism. For the first time, my wife Kay and I understood what it meant to be parents of a child with special needs. This was when I realized that I was terribly wrong in my understanding of individuals with special needs.

Mark taught us many amazing and wonderful things. Because of Mark, I was able to become a children's pastor at a large church in Kansas City. God then lead me to Grace Church in Overland Park, Kansas, where I started the SOAR (Special, Opportunities, Abilities, and Relationships) Special Needs Ministry and am now the SOAR Special Needs Pastor.

Mark was cured of his Dravet syndrome and autism on November 1, 2010, when he was born into heaven at the age of five and a half. Kay and I were blessed to be Mark's parents! God used Mark's time here on earth with us to teach us and prepare us to be able to minister now to hundreds of other families and to walk alongside them, through the highs and the lows.

During Mark's short time on earth, we always held him to the same disciplinary standards that we do our other kids and we would always encourage him to do things he hadn't done before. SOAR was created seven months after Mark's death, and it was a couple of years before I realized that SOAR is part of Mark's ausome potential! Because Mark is in heaven, and because God blessed my family with him, today I am passionate for families with special needs and work endlessly to minister to them, which fills me with complete joy. I am living out Mark's purpose!

SOAR Special Needs Ministry is Mark's legacy and potential. As of August 2017, SOAR currently ministers to over 650 individuals with special needs of all ages and severities and we have also assisted over 150 churches from all over the country in starting or improving their special needs ministries. Because of Mark, God has given us the vision to help develop 1000 special needs ministries in churches throughout the world in the next twenty years! Mark's ausome potential is being a major Kingdom builder.

Whether you are a parent or you are working in a special needs ministry, know that every individual with special needs has *ausome potential*! Never just settle, always challenge your child to become the absolute best that they can be! Help them to dream and then help them to accomplish that dream! One of our students is an extremely talented artist; growing up, her parents always encouraged her to draw and to use her imagination. As a result, my great friend, Catlaina Vrana, nineteen years old, is now a published author and illustrator! She has written and illustrated two books and is currently working on her third! Her second book, *Ella Autie: A Book About Autism Written by an Autistic Person*, gives great insight into the mind of an individual with autism. Catlaina has *ausome potential*! On top of that, she is also a very gifted pianist and singer. She is even able to sing in multiple languages! Today she is an amazing self-advocate for individuals with autism. She is using her ausome potential to influence others.

If you are a ministry leader, you can tap into your students' ausome potential and combine it with ministry! Andrew is sixteen years old and has Down syndrome and loves to work with younger children and to help others. He serves every Sunday in our kindergarten room. He stands at the door and greets all of the parents and kids with a high five or fist bump and then his job is to prepare the snacks while the class is in worship. It is pure joy to watch Andrew serve others every week. Emmitt is eighteen years old and has autism; he loves music and kids. As we got to know Emmitt and his family, we learned that he is passionate about doing the actions to the music. Now Emmitt works with our Vacation Bible School and our actioneers team and he assists with leading everyone in learning the actions to the songs for VBS. It is so incredible to watch both Andrew and Emmitt applying their ausome potential in the church setting as they are now using it to become Kingdom builders! Don't miss out on this very special level of Kingdom building in your ministry!

So, parents and leaders, how can you help your child with special needs reach their ausome potential? First, observe your child and see what interests them. Next, make an effort to be supportive and positive to your child. Make sure they hear you say "Good job," "I'm proud of you!" or "That is awesome!" Avoid negative comments; instead encourage them in realizing that they can do whatever their dream is. One way you can do this is exposing them to new things, which helps pique their curiosity which in turn increases their desire to learn. Studies show that children with autism learn faster, stay focused longer, and are generally better behaved when they are regularly challenged with fun new tasks. This can be accomplished by going on outings or "field trips" to new places and seeing interesting things that can start conversations and jumpstart the imagination and their desire to learn more. Turn everyday events into learning opportunities, encouraging your child to explore and ask questions.

Allow your child to teach you through different mediums, especially if they are nonverbal! Encourage them to communicate through music, art, acting, writing, or dancing. These are all great ways for them to express themselves and great opportunities for them to show their ausome potential! Play therapy is another great way to promote self-expression, as well as reading books with your child, which for many can open some wonderful adventures and create some new passions for your child.

If your child has an interest in learning something new, you can assist them without adding extra pressure or setting them up for failure.

Keep it simple. Find ways to informally encourage your child's interest. Get some fun songs on CD or karaoke and have fun singing; or borrow an instrument and let them play on it, showing them how to place their hands or play some notes. Get some copy paper and start doodling or sketching with crayons, pencils, or even finger paints with your child and see what develops. Put on your own dance performance in your living room with the music playing. Pick up a basketball and shoot baskets, play catch, or kick a soccer ball around in the backyard.

Get lessons. If your child continues to show interest, start looking for a tutor or instructor who has experience or is comfortable working with a child with special needs. There are great clubs for the sports like Miracle League, Challenger Sports, and Special Olympics. Your city may have special dance troops, theater/acting groups, or cheer teams for individuals with special needs.

Keep it fun! Don't pressure your child to meet specific goals or to practice constantly. Instead, focus on only giving positive feedback for their effort. Give fun rewards for them meeting their goals or practice time (anything from time on the iPad to a special treat, whatever your child considers a fun incentive). Try changing the atmosphere or location for the practice—move it outside, into a different room, or do it by candle light. This can keep the experience fresh and fun. Do whatever you can to prevent the practice time from becoming boring.

Praise the activity! Whenever your child does the activity, praise them for it, especially if they show enjoyment! Be patient and keep in mind that these skills don't come overnight. If your child doesn't practice every day, that is fine! Don't push them and make them not enjoy it. Allow them to enjoy it and build their passion for it. As their passion grows, they will naturally want to do it more!

Most importantly, remember that God has given your child specific skills and talents. Ephesians 2:10 says, "For we are God's masterpiece. He has created us anew in Christ Jesus, so we can do the good things He planned for us long ago" (NLT). The Greek word for "masterpiece" is *poema*, the word we get "poem" from. God is saying we are his poem, we are his masterpiece. He has designed you and your children with gifts—passions, abilities, experiences, and personalities. God designed your child to enjoy the things they like to do. This doesn't say everyone but those with special needs, nor does it say only certain people; it says "we," meaning every single individual! Embrace this and remember God has given every single person special skills and talents that he desires for us to use for his good and his purposes. How cool is that! God has given every single one of our kids *ausome potential*! It is our job as parents and ministry leaders to help unearth that potential and to grow it into its maximum potential, and who knows what legacy that could bring!

Now what do you see when you see an individual with special needs? I encourage you to view a video that our SOAR Special Needs Ministry developed called "I See." You can find it on the SOAR Special Needs Ministry YouTube page. We took several individuals in our ministry and asked them what they see when they view themselves in a mirror. My question is, what do you see? I hope you see *ausome potential*! My prayer is that you ask God to help you to find your child's *ausome potential* and that you will have the wisdom and discernment to know how to help groom your child in developing it.

•••

AUSOME THOUGHTS

When God says you are his masterpiece, nothing can hold you back from your potential, not even a disability. We really can't even imagine all the plans that God has for these differently-abled individuals. Only God knows the scope of how he will use each story and the legacy that each life will leave. The ausome potential is there and we have only to look to the one who created us to fulfill that destiny. "What no eye has seen, nor ear heard, nor the heart of man imagined, what God has prepared for those who love him" (2 Cor. 2:9). Dream *big*, because we can't even imagine how he will use our ausome blessings!

—Beth

chapter 8

Ausome Community

by Sandra Robinson

High Speed, Low Drag

TODAY WE CELEBRATED THE LIFE of one of our family's greatest joys: my uncle Butch. He was my mom's youngest brother, eight years my senior, and I can't remember a time when he wasn't part of my life. Butch was blind and developmentally delayed. He left behind very few material things. Though he didn't have a plethora of friends, those who knew him were significantly impacted by his life. I firmly believe that, besides Jesus Christ, Butch has been the most influential individual regarding the trajectory and scope of the ministry that God has called me to.

Butch taught me about God's character and how he views individuals with special needs, or Champions. All exceptional individuals are Champions because they must overcome so many obstacles to live healthy, productive lives. Many of the things that are marginalized in this world are the very things that are highly valued and honored in the Kingdom of God. "Listen, my beloved brethren: Has God not chosen the poor of this world *to be* rich in faith and heirs of the kingdom which He promised to those who love Him?" (Jas. 2:5, NKJV). Butch was considered a poor man by the world's standards. He was labelled by others as being financially, intellectually, mentally, and spiritually poor. But the opposite was true: He was a rich man. He owned real estate in God's Kingdom. According to the Bible, Butch has a mansion in heaven.

He had a remarkable memory and could tell you what was said about you while you weren't there. This talent caused many of us to rethink what we said about others, especially when Butch was around. He loved God and enjoyed Christmas music because it reminded him of God's love. Christmas carols could be heard booming from his bedroom any day at any time.

All individuals, regardless of their abilities, are handcrafted by God and made in his image, and Butch was uniquely formed by God. He was God's masterpiece. "For we are His workmanship, created in Christ Jesus for good works, which God prepared beforehand that we should walk in them" (Eph. 2:10, NKJV). Exceptional individuals aren't cursed or a result of sin, but are with us to show us God's glory. "Now as [Jesus] passed by, He saw a man who was blind from birth. And His disciples asked Him, saying, 'Rabbi, who sinned, this man or his parents, that he was born blind?' Jesus answered, 'Neither this man nor his parents sinned, but that the works of God should be revealed in him'" (John 9:1-3, NKJV).

Every individual has a purpose. Our purpose is to come to know and love God and to share his love with others. It has been my experience that God often uses the ausomely blessed to soften the hearts of those around them so they can experience God's love. It's God's will that exceptional individuals be members of God's family. His family is complete when all his creation is together, connected to each other so we can fulfill our purpose. "In the same way, even though we are many individuals, Christ makes us one body and individuals who are connected to each other" (Rom. 12:5, GW).

We are all one family, one flock, with one purpose, and we can learn a lot by observing the wonders of God's creations. Years ago a pair of Canadian geese laid their eggs in the planter right outside my classroom door. My students and I were fascinated by them. We fed them, protected them, and gave them names. I was so enthralled with these animals that my students gave me the moniker of "Mother Goose." We eagerly found out all we could about these amazing creatures. We learned that geese mate for life, lay about five or six eggs in the spring, and the female incubates the eggs for twenty-five to thirty days. Their young are called goslings and at only ten weeks old they can fly. Geese migrate in flocks to warmer climates in the winter months. As we continued to gather facts about these amazing animals, I began to see many similarities between their behavior and our journey with Butch.

Geese fly in a V formation, which provides each individual goose with a cohesive community with direction and purpose, a way to communicate wants and needs, and a comprehensive care plan. A community is a group that shares a common interest, identity, and purpose. Driven by instinct, the geese are compelled to fly to warmer climates in the winter where they can find the resources needed to sustain life and the species. Traveling in the V formation requires each goose to make a contribution to reach the destination. Each goose flapping its wings in the formation creates uplift and reduces the drag or wind resistance for the bird immediately behind it. The greater the drag, the more energy the goose must expound to fly. Reducing drag increases flight efficiency. Flying in a V formation allows the flock to travel seventy percent farther with the same energy than if each goose flew alone.

"High speed, low drag" is a military term that means the mission can be achieved with optimum precision and efficiency so that no additional support is needed. This is comparable to when the goose has reached the sweet spot in the formation where it is able to fly at its greatest speed with the least amount of effort because there is little or no resistance. High speed, low drag can only be achieved if each goose is willing to remain in formation and take its turn as the windcutter.

There is always a leader, or what some call a windcutter, while geese are in flight. This is a difficult, but vital job. The windcutter's position is at the vertex of the V formation. All other geese form two lines fanning out behind the windcutter. It is responsible for breaking up the flow of air for the flock. This windcutter expends the greatest amount of energy because it makes the initial cut through the wind and experiences the greatest amount of resistance. These extreme conditions make it physically impossible for one goose to be a windcutter for the entire flight, so they take turns. In order for the flock to remain in flight for as long as possible, an exhausted windcutter will drop out of the leadership position and move to the rear of the formation, where the resistance is lightest, and another goose will take its turn in the windcutter position.

Like the flock of migrating geese, those of us who have loved ones with special needs are on a long journey. When we fly solo, fatigue can easily set in and deter us from continuing our flight. We are more successful in arriving at our destination when we fly with our community, remain in formation, and take our turn being a windcutter.

Butch was our windcutter throughout my childhood, and he taught me so much. Butch flew with amazing grace and power as he showed me who he was and how exceptional individuals must be accepted, respected, and given their place in the formation. When I became a young adult, it was my turn to be a windcutter. I was Butch's advocate, caregiver, protector, teacher, and friend. Then I became a windcutter for the ever growing families God has put into our formation. There have been many times when I have felt the fatigue of the position. At those times God has provided new windcutters to lead our flock.

Lizzy is one of the truly inspiring windcutters of our flock. She and her husband Isaac love the Lord and each other and serve as amazing, highly effective pastors at a church in Northern California. They have two incredible boys: Noah and Calvin. Their younger son, Calvin, was diagnosed as having autism.

Upon receiving this news, Lizzy, like most parents, was devastated. She wanted to isolate herself and her family from the world, and wondered, "Why me, God?" She was thrown onto an emotional roller coaster as she began to advocate for her child in the precarious world of special education. At that time the farthest thing from Lizzy's mind was ministering to others, but God called her to do just that. Even though she felt physically, emotionally, mentally, and sometimes spiritually depleted, she decided to minister to others who were going through similar struggles. She allowed God to turn the trials of her family into opportunities for her to share her faith. Lizzy began to see that God was using her experiences to spread the gospel and allow others to encounter his unfailing love and care. She is living Philippians 1:12 daily: "But I want you to know brethren, that the things which happened to me have actually turned out for the furtherance of the Gospel" (NKJV). God used her fearless and relentless quest to obtain resources for her son and others to bring hope and empower other caregivers to rise up and be advocates for the individuals with a disability in their community. In other words, Lizzy became a powerful, masterful windcutter, who in turn encouraged others to take their positions as windcutters. Being a windcutter, though challenging at times, has given Lizzy amazing joy and fulfillment.

The V formation of a flock of geese in flight allows for optimum communication, even when they face challenges. In this formation, the loud, show-stopping honks of geese can easily be heard by all members of the flock. These honks provide each goose with identity, direction, and encouragement to keep up with the flock. The honks let the flock know when danger is present and when and where to stop to feed and rest. Some scientists say that the jarring honk of a goose is its expression of pure joy and excitement over the ability to fly with their community. Just like the flock of geese, communication in our community is vital. Often, our ausomely blessed require a variety of resources to enable them to reach their individual destiny in Christ and remain in the formation. We learn from each other and outside agencies how to best minister to our Champions so they stay with the flock.

One of the greatest strengths of the V formation is that it provides the flock with the capability to care for its members. Researchers have discovered that when one goose becomes weak, ill, or injured and drops out of the formation, two other geese fall out of formation and remain with their fellow traveler until it is able to fly again or dies. Many people did this for us. When our family was struggling to find answers regarding Butch's care, many people helped us, encouraged us, and just listened to us. Their care and support allowed us to heal and join the flock once more.

There are many ways to be a windcutter for the individuals with a disability and their families. We can provide moral support by listening to their struggles without judgment, inviting them to social functions, and providing a safe place for them to go during difficult times. We can donate our time by providing respite care, attending their Individual Education Plan meetings, or going with Champions to their doctor or dentist appointments. When Champions or their loved ones are sick or pass away, we can demonstration our compassion for them by being with them during their time of greatest need. We can remind them that we are all part of God's flock and they are not alone.

Since I was a small girl, Butch has been the windcutter God gave me to set me on the path he wanted me to walk down for the rest of my life. Butch taught me to be a fierce advocate, patient teacher, and loving friend to the exceptional members of our flock and their families. I will see you soon in heaven, Butch, and I hope you will smile at me and say, "You travelled at high speed with low drag. Welcome home." Until that day, I will take my place in the formation and keep honking.

• • •

AUSOME THOUGHTS

God never intended us to do life alone. It is part of his design that we live in community. Hebrews 10:24-25 says, "And let us consider how to stir up one another to love and good works, not neglecting to meet together, as is the habit of some, but encouraging one another, and all the more as you see the Day drawing near." I pray that each person reading this book feels themselves surrounded by an ausome community of love and support. If not, I encourage you to bravely step out and be that community to someone else. It's amazing the network that God will build through one ausomely connected individual!

—Beth

chapter 9

We Love Luci

Stories of how God shows up miraculously in the everyday and has brought friends, healing, and peace through the community he has built around our ausome blessing, Luci.

I'M SO THANKFUL THAT I had the pleasure of working with and getting to know Miss Luci. She quickly became a dear part of my life and her laughter and energy will always be contagious! I truly miss working with her but am so proud of how far she's come and what a lovely young lady she is—I know her family and friends just adore her!

One of my favorite memories of Luci is riding on her four-wheeler outside as she cheered me on. She loved that thing! (I'm guessing she still does? Haha!)

Another funny tidbit is that she burst into laughter any time she went through the alphabet and landed on the letter "F." We had worked on pronunciation of the letter "F" at one point and she laughed every time she said it. I'll never forget that. Haha! Luci is one amazing gal!

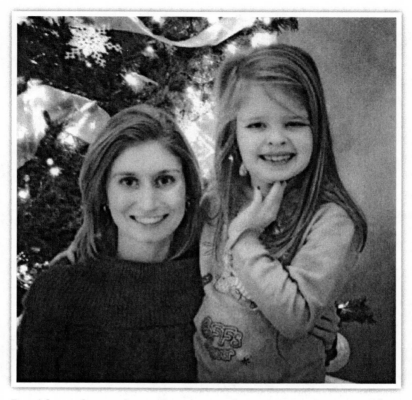

Luci has always brought so much joy, right from the start. Luci, I remember the day your mom told me you would be coming soon. You were a miracle from the beginning. Then you decided to arrive a bit early and caught me out of town.

I remember the first time I heard you laugh. It was as someone was pouring glass rocks into a vase, which apparently was hysterical. Not much has changed; loud and somewhat disruptive things are still super funny!

I love you, Luci and all you bring to our lives—like humility. For instance, the time we were at the mall with your mom but you and I were in line together. You were probably around seven and in a phase of hitting or pushing people as a hello. There was an elderly lady in front of us and with no warning you smacked her right on the backside. And, of course, smiled your little smile. She turned and seemed genuinely confused with which one of us was the culprit. I didn't clarify for her but looked over at your mom as she was in the line beside us and tried to decide if I should melt into the floor or burst out laughing. Your mom, by the way, seemed super content to let me take the heat that particular day and did not indicate in any way that she was with us. Never a dull moment.

After all the prayers for your speech, I love how much you love to hear yourself talk. (Or let's be real, you love to hear yourself yell.) On the train ride at the zoo a few summers ago, you got to say, "All aboard" and took full advantage of the microphone projected over the loud speaker. Pretty sure that "all aboard" was heard miles from the zoo. Thinking of that story and many others, I am grateful because you bring our family even closer together, I think. I remember each face when you made the "all aboard" announcement. We (aunts, uncles, and grandparents) were all grinning from ear to ear and chuckling as we knew how much you loved doing that.

I suppose I could go on and on. I am very grateful that God has blessed me with having the opportunity to be a part of Luci's life.

—Abby Koontz

Okay, here is my Luci story. Me, my sister Alyssa, and my friend Corinne have been working during first service of our church in the kindergarten through sixth grade class with my dad. I love every Sunday coming downstairs and seeing Luci run over to sit by all us leaders. She loves to just sit there, flip through her Bible, ask for Skittles, and scream "Corinnneeeeee!" really loud. Anyway, one particular Sunday my dad, Mr. Matt, asked the classroom what they wanted the next Sunday for breakfast. They could ask for anything and he would make it. Some kids asked for biscuits and gravy, others asked for pancakes, a few said doughnuts, but Luci wanted Pop-Tarts. She raised her hand

and yelled, "Mr. Matt, I want Pop-Tarts!" My dad said okay and moved on. Later after the kids had voted, he announced that he was going bring pancakes and doughnuts. All of the sudden Luci screamed, "No!" and put her head down. I tried to ask Luci what was wrong, but she just kept saying no. Finally at the end of class, my dad came up to Luci, and he asked her what was wrong. She said, "Mr. Matt, are you mad at me?" He responded with, "Luci, why would I be mad at you?" I then connected the dots and realized what the problem was. Once I passed along this message to my dad, he responded, "Luci, I'll get you Pop-Tarts next week, okay?" She then lifted her head, grabbed my arm, and had the biggest grin on her face. Luci will always bring so much joy to my life and love to my heart. I love you, Luci!

—Lexi Carmichael

I am often brought to tears when thinking back to the time I got to spend working with Luci in Awana. That was the stage where she was beginning to break out of that nonverbal world she was stuck in. At the start of the year, she could usually repeat one word at a time for her verses; sometimes I couldn't keep her focused long enough for that, though. The whole class would start to do it that way so that she would, often without prompting. Each week, she would stand with all the other girls and get her jewels. Those girls loved being with her and working alongside her! They saw no barriers. As the weeks went on, Luci started showing signs that she was more and more in tune with what was going on and that she wanted to be a part of it. Eventually, we started doing phrase by phrase with verses—and then we started doing just about the whole verse all at once! Week by week she would surprise me with each new accomplishment and improvement. Luci was there—and she was fighting her way to the surface. Watching her break out of that world on the inside and into the world of relationships has always brought a smile to my face! To remember that little Luci, and to look at her now, I stand in awe of God's love and faithfulness, and I am thankful that he gave not only Ryan and Beth the opportunity to love Luci, but he chose to give our church family a little extra blessing when he created her!

—Brittany Russell

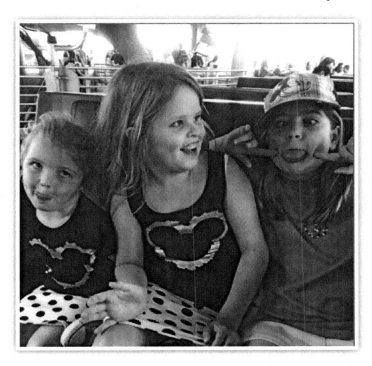

I've known Luci for about four years. She's a wonderful friend! I remember the first time I met her, I heard there was going to be a new student at our school. A couple of days later I met Luci at recess. Then after a while, I played with Luci about every day. I got to know Luci better in the fourth grade. I met her parents, and I was also in the same class with her that year. Autism will never stop me from being her friend, and it will never stop Luci from being herself.

—Saralyn Pendleton

I think my favorite story of Luci was from a couple years ago during the *Alive* performance. One child was having a melt-down and his father (who was playing the part of Jesus) heard him from the welcome center area. The boy's father came into the children's area, where we were, to talk to his son. This Dad was in full costume when he came back there. I didn't think much of it until Luci started talking. "Jesus? Jesus?! *Jesus*?! Myanna, I be good, okay? Myanna, I be good, okay?!" Luci will sometimes try me to see what she can get away with, but after Jesus appeared to talk to the boy, there was no trying me at all that night!

—Marlanna Swanson

Luci's love is amazing! She is never ashamed to hug me and love me in public. Her love is never a put-on or for show. It is one hundred percent authentic. She is always so happy to be with me in my truck or just sit on my lap. Loving her back is so easy. I'm so thankful that the Lord has given us such a perfect and precious gift.

—Perry Frank (Pappaw Perry)

In my world autism has a name and that name is Luci and I love her so much! When she was very young and we were finding out the challenges that she was facing, I remember one day sitting in her little special needs classroom and fighting back the tears thinking that this doesn't seem fair to Luci to have such challenges. Her parents being in full-time ministry, I felt like it wasn't fair. As the years have gone on and I've been able to see how her parents, my son and daughter-in-law, have now included special needs as part of their ministry, I see God's hand in the whole thing. I see all the lessons that Luci has taught us! Through her life she has affected each one of us, her little cousins, her aunts and uncles, and me as her grandma. I now realize that the challenge that Luci faces is a mysterious amazing gift that is teaching each one of us so many lessons and growing us into a deeper walk with God. Luci has a walk with God that is so pure and so beautiful and I am so blessed to be her grandma. God has taught me through the life of my beautiful granddaughter Luci that even when we face challenges, we can trust a loving faithful God that has seen the whole picture and knows the blessing that have come from this challenge, and that blessing and gift in my life is Luci.

—Judy Frank (Mammaw Judy)

Tower, elevated, great light.

I was there the day you all were getting ready to leave the hospital. Ryan told me the choice of names you were considering. When he said Madeline Lucille, it's hard to explain my feeling, but it just clicked. "That is perfect for her," I thought. At this time, we didn't know the challenges you and she would face in life. Our prayers for your new family were many.

Some years later after finding out she had autism, the Lord woke me in the middle of the night. I was to pray for her and you all. With tears streaming, I poured out my heart on her behalf. The prayers have continued but never again with this intensity was I prompted to pray. As I remember this night and the years of concern and struggle, I am overjoyed at where the Lord has taken you because of Madeline Lucille. Through your experiences and God's faithfulness, God is erecting a magnificent tower of light to encourage and help others.

Luci is like a beacon in a lighthouse. Though the way may be rough and at times a torment of storms, she is a bright light in the midst and draws others to Jesus, the true light.

Madeline means: tower, elevated, great. Lucille means: light. Luci was well named, Mom and Dad, well named.

— Aunt Marian (Marian Rickner)

I love Luci!! I remember the first couple of weeks that Luci started to come down stairs for Junior Church. I would put games together for Elizabeth's lesson and Luci was so interested in everything I was doing. She would talk to me and ask me questions. I just remember being so determined after that for Luci to like me and be my friend. I sat by her that day, talked to her, and told her my name. The next week I came back to junior church not expecting her to remember, but right as I got downstairs I hear her yell, "CORINNE!!!!!" and get excited for me to be there. To this day, if I'm not sitting by her and she sees me, she will yell my name! Luci never fails to put a smile on my face. Even when she licks me every time she sees me! She always tells me "that was gross, I'm sorry Corinne. I love you!" She is very determined too! Whenever I am with her, she is very persistent that Lexi and Alyssa have to be there too. That girl knows what she wants!

—Corinne Walker

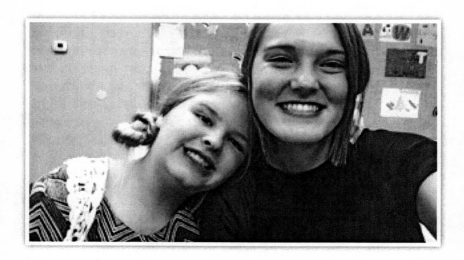

chapter 10

Ausome Faith

by Barb Newman

My body has autism but my spirit does not.
—Teen with Autism Spectrum Disorder from Michigan

Once a year we offer 'worship and wiggles,' which is a time
when we encourage our children to stand up and worship and
move as they wish. While we had been including a child with
autism spectrum disorder in worship, he rarely participated
in any visible way. But on this day, he took the lead. He stood
up and started to move and dance. We could see how he was
connecting with God in worship and it inspired the other
children to move and it moved the adults to tears. I think we
will be offering this option way more than once a year. He was a
worship leader on this day.
—Children's Ministry Director from Kentucky

Our congregation had to learn what worship is about from a
youth with autism spectrum disorder. It was his turn to serve as
an acolyte. (An acolyte in this church is anyone who performs
a ceremonial duty such as lighting altar candles.) People did
not think he could or should do this as he had no ability to speak

and would often just run around the church. But on this day, he picked up the unlit candle and started to run with it around the congregation. As he encircled the people, it became clear that he was performing this role in a way that beautifully added to the worship experience. God used him powerfully in this role, and we will continue to have him take his turn as a worship leader.
—Pastor from New York City

Our group was discussing Good Friday and Easter. As I was telling the story, a young girl with Down syndrome was in tears with the events of that Friday. Then I told the part about the resurrection. The other children got caught up in the celebration as the girl started to dance and celebrate like she was at a huge party. Her joy was contagious and undoubtedly a sweet offering to the Lord.
—Sunday school teacher from Seattle

Perspective

After thirty plus years of teaching and leading groups that include children with disabilities, I praise God for the seat he has given me—the seat in the front row to watch his work in the lives of individuals and inclusive groups. The four stories and quotes above are only a drop in the bucket of what I have learned from the words and actions of children of varied abilities and disabilities. What a view I have had! I want to share with you a few of the things God has shown me about the faith life of individuals with disabilities and the impact that faith has had on the family, friends, and community around that person.

Lesson 1: Jesus used accommodations and we need to follow suit.

If there was a five-star rating system for the way Jesus taught, he would earn all five stars! Jesus would teach to large groups, small groups, and sometimes one-on-one. He would use illustrations that were meaningful to those he taught, and he would frequently tell stories so people could understand his main point. He would place challenges before people as well as encouragement. He could teach people who were sitting, boating, walking, or standing. He captured the experience of the moment, or created experiences, to bring a point home. Remember those nets full of fish after a very dry spell of fishing? Also, Jesus knew those he was speaking to so well, the woman at the well said in John 4:29 to the people of her town, "Come, see a man who told me everything I ever did." Jesus was a five-star teacher partly because he knew the audience and came up with experiences and learning that would allow each one to grow and understand.

We need to use Jesus as our model when we introduce Jesus to any child, but especially a child with unique gifts and needs. We need to begin by knowing that child. What makes that person smile and what does that individual love to do? While it is sometimes easy to think about the person's limitations, I would challenge you to consider that child's gifts and strengths. What can this person do? If this person best relates to pictures, then get some pictures that tell the story of Jesus. If this person loves to move, then set up a way to move from station to station as you explore the salvation story. If the individual loves a particular book or movie, find ways to have those characters explain the love of Jesus for the child.

My book *Accessible Gospel, Inclusive Worship* (Barbara J. Newman, CLC Network: 2015) offers many additional suggestions and stories that will help you come up with a plan especially chosen for the individual(s) in your life. As I note on page 19, "Instead of shoving this person into a 'one size fits all' curriculum or class, let's design supports around this person so we can best reach and include this friend, child, sibling, or aging parent."

Lesson 2: Everyone deserves to grow in their faith. We share ownership in making that happen.

Family devotions, individual times with God, Sunday school, and corporate worship are all examples of the ways many of us choose to continue to grow and learn. Yet, I have heard countless stories from families that it has been challenging to find a place of worship for every family member. Asked to leave, assigned the job of "buddy" to their own child, or simply ignored or ostracized, families frequently have difficulty finding access to some of the key places and events that allow us each to grow in Christ.

Church communities, consider this a reminder to look at your options and make sure you have created a welcoming place for people of all abilities. Did you plan Sunday school expecting children with varied abilities to attend? Do you have options for children with shorter attention spans or unique sensory systems? Are your volunteers and leaders equipped and ready to engage with each child in their group? Do you have a plan in place or a process to follow when a visiting family attends and one of the children may have autism spectrum disorder?

There are so many, many supports available to you. A great place to begin is to think about the role you play in your church community; be assured that there are things you can do to welcome and include each one. From the person purchasing products for the bathrooms to the individual picking up snack items to the worship leader or small group leader, jump right in. CLC Network has created a great tool to help you look up your role and suggest items for you to consider. Visit clcnetwork.org/for-churches/roles/ to get started.

Parents, consider this an opportunity to look at your posture. I can guarantee that your child will bring gifts and opportunities to a church community that they have not yet imagined. God has gifted each one of his children with gifts to grow the body. Your child's absence is a loss; your child's presence is a gift. Please don't approach church leadership with your head down, guilty look on your face, and ask, "Please, maybe, do you have any spot for my child with, um, Down syndrome?" I have often challenged parents to approach leadership and say, "Have I got a deal for you!" While those may not be your exact words, consider the opportunities for the congregation as you make arrangements for Sunday school, youth group, or Wednesday night kid's club.

Lesson 3: "As it is, there are many parts, but one body." (1 Cor. 12: 20)

I have learned so very, very much from interacting and living in community with persons with disabilities. While some churches believe there needs to be a "special program" or "special treasures room" for any child with a disability, I can assure you that we all benefit from learning and growing together. While there may need to be accommodations, planning, and support, giving children options to be part of the same group with varied abilities will offer a chance for everyone to share their gifts. Doing all we can to keep the body of Christ together grows communities of people who acknowledge that God has handcrafted each person with unique gifts and needs, yet we need each other to be whole and complete.

My friend Adam blessed so many people in his lifetime. He was passionate in worship, often asking others present to join in. He was also a servant. Adam enjoyed vacuuming and yard work, and often used those gifts to serve aging neighbors or the well-carpeted church building. Adam's life also showed some of the unique qualities expected in a person with Down syndrome and autism spectrum disorder—the two disabilities he lived with. Yet, Adam's parents were confident that he needed to grow and learn in the heart of the community with other individuals his age. The testimony to this truth was evident at his memorial service. We were expecting perhaps a hundred people, as this was one of two settings to remember Adam. Five hundred people showed up that night, and those who spoke never once mentioned Down syndrome or ASD! They did, however, mention how God has used Adam to teach and to touch their lives. Adam and his five hundred plus friends are one example of many. Preserve the body, live life together, and learn from one another. (You can read more of Adam's story in *I Choose Adam: Nothing Special Please,* written by his father David Winstrom, 2017.)

• • •

AUSOME THOUGHTS

The simple words and strong faith of children with disabilities have a profound effect because they speak straight from heaven.

There is a saying: "It doesn't have to be perfect to be beautiful." In the case of ausome faith, I would say that being imperfect makes it more beautiful according to 2 Corinthians 11:30: "If I must boast, I will boast of the things that show my weakness." What is more beautiful than grace in action?! God wants authentic service and worship in his Kingdom and welcomes it. He is intentionally building the body of Christ with varied abilities and disabilities working together in unity. Each member of the body has a specific purpose and there is a need for each and every member to be doing exactly what they were designed to do. Because of their simple words and strong faith, children with special needs have a profound effect. How the world would change if we could all have ausome faith!

—Beth

chapter 11

Ausome Friendship

by Norma Puga

I T'S NEVER GOD'S INTENT THAT we walk through this life alone. He has ordained special people to develop special friendships that are a blessing both to the special needs child and the special friend. I believe that it takes someone very special and with a beautiful heart to want to reach out and begin a relationship. These individuals have to be able to see ausome kids as people with abilities instead of someone with a disability. They have to be able to take the time to cultivate and nurture the relationship. They have to be able to enter their world and to see them as the people God created them to be. They have to be able to look them in the eyes and see that they too have a purpose in this life. They also have to be the ones who start giving the most in the relationship.

I have heard ausome kids described as children behind a thin veil. I believe that it is our job to go through that veil and reach them. We should not expect them to be able to step into our world.

Jeremiah 29:11 says, "'For I know the plans I have for you,' declares the Lord, 'plans to prosper you and not to harm you, plans to give you hope and a future.'" This scripture is intended for these individuals as well. You may be called to be part of that plan. You may be called to help them understand what God's plan is for them. Do not pass up the opportunity to befriend them.

To begin to establish a relationship with someone with special needs takes time. You have to begin to earn their trust and confidence. You have to be there with them through their roughest moments and be able to accept them for who they are. You cannot be judgmental and take anything personally. You have to learn how they communicate and know that they were created with gifts and talents like everyone else. You have the unique opportunity to search out and see what their special gifts and talents are. You have to learn what their level of understanding is and be able to meet them there. You have to make the commitment and stay in it for the long haul. It is a love journey that you begin and when it blossoms into a relationship, it is an extraordinary feeling that is difficult to describe.

It is very easy to befriend and come to love a person with special needs. They are so pure in heart and there are never any hidden agendas. What you see is what you get. It is a pure, genuine, and simple relationship. I have had the opportunity to work with so many children, teens, and adults on all levels of the spectrum and I have been able to witness many types of these relationships.

In my many years of working at Lakewood Church alongside these children, teens, and adults with special needs, many of the relationships formed have been between the volunteer and the child. Volunteers who commit to serving in a special needs ministry often join thinking that they are there to bless someone. After a while they realize that they were the ones who ended up with the blessings. The heart has been given, the relationship is formed, and the attachment is strong. Most of these relationships were not intentional. They just happened out of the time that they were able to spend together. One of my volunteers says that God speaks to her through her special relationship. She often tells me that when she is having a hard day or week and she sees her little guy, one hug from him and she knows that God is there. She feels God's presence and that helps her get through the rest of the week. That is her "love-bug" and there is nothing she wouldn't do for him. She gets pure joy from seeing and being around him. I know that her life has been enriched because of that relationship.

There have been a few relationships that have been formed between the individuals with special needs. It is a beautiful relationship and it is awesome to see the development of these friendships. There is one friendship that has developed between two of our teens with special needs in our program. It is so wonderful to see this friendship flourish between these two young men. It began quite simply with them asking each other questions on what their likes and dislikes were. They would get into intense conversations about their favorite topics. In the months that pursued, that relationship grew closer and stronger and they looked forward to seeing each other each week. They began to communicate by phone during the week. When one of them graduated from high school, he had to make sure that his friend was a part of that. They hung out together after the graduation. They are best friends. For the parents this was a dream come true. Each one of the boys struggled to make friends at school but when they would arrive at church, they would be so focused on each other and interacted on their level. Merriam-Webster defines friend as "one attached to another by affection or esteem." I believe these two formed an attachment to each other based on the fact that there was no judgment on either of their sides. They accepted each other as they were and felt comfortable around each other.

Since most teens with special needs lack the socialization skills needed to foster any type of relationship, it is difficult for them to know how to begin a relationship. They want to be accepted by society and their peers, yet they do not know where to begin. It is very important that we all take the time and begin helping them cope in our world.

First Corinthians 12:27 says, "Now you are the body of Christ and each one of you is a part of it." We have to realize that they too have a part in our lives. It is our responsibility to get involved and help them navigate through this life and the only way we can do this is to begin a relationship with one of them.

We can learn so many things from them. One of the things that I personally have learned from them is humility. There is never any pride or arrogance in them. I can see their goodness and innocence. My tank fills up after I have spent time with them. I too believed that I was going to be a blessing to these families, but in turn I was the one who received the blessing. It is a joy that I cannot get anywhere else. I consider it an honor that God has chosen me to be a part of this special community.

In Matthew 25:40 Jesus says, "Truly I tell you, whatever you did for one of the least of these brothers and sisters of mine, you did for me. I believe that through these individuals Jesus is giving us the perfect opportunity to be his hands and feet. We should seek ways to be a part of their community. Get involved in organizations that service or work with children, teens, or adults with special needs.

We may never know until we get to heaven the real impact that was made on the individual. If they are not verbal or have difficulty communicating, they may not be able to fully express or communicate how they feel or what your friendship means to them. But I know that God will find a way to let you know that he is pleased with what you are doing. Every effort that you make toward establishing a relationship will be paid back. You may not understand the effect you are having in their lives, but all the deposits that you make into their lives will be rewarded.

In Mark 10:14 Jesus says, "Let the little children come to me, and do not hinder them, for the kingdom of God belongs to such as these." I often think of them as God's angels sent down to help me learn and grow in the way that I should treat everyone. They have helped me become a better person. I have learned to celebrate them for who they are. I know that God has given me the amazing opportunity to lift them up and to speak positive words over their lives. I do not take for granted that I get to be a part of their lives if only for a short amount of time each week.

Let us not waste the opportunity to seek out these individuals and engage them in a relationship. They can enrich your life immensely. Do not pass up the chance to be a part of their lives and help develop them into the people God created them to be.

• • •

AUSOME THOUGHTS

Ausome friendship is possible! God has answered so many of the prayers I have prayed for Luci and one of the biggest ways was bringing her beautiful friendships. As you can tell by reading the "We Love Luci" chapters, our girl has a whole community of love and support around her #teamluci. God built that! We have met the most unexpected people and formed connections that will last a lifetime because of our ausome blessing! God even arranged for one of Luci's closest friends from school to be at Disney World the very same day as our family so that they could go on rides together—what an unexpected blessing! How our heavenly Father loves us and works out all the details, small and large, including bringing along some ausome friends to lighten the load and bring a smile to our hearts. ☺

—Beth

chapter 12

Ausome Ministers

by Sandra Peoples

T HE DAYS AFTER PARENTS HEAR their child has a disability or special need can be difficult days. Most parents go through a mourning process. The expectations and dreams they may have had for their child die and new ones must take root. Some are in a whirlwind of doctor's appointments. Some feel like they are learning a new language of acronyms and medical terms. All of them need an anchor to help steady them. Their church should be that anchor that reminds them God is in control and has a plan for them and their entire family.

My husband is a pastor, so when our son got an autism diagnosis in 2010, we couldn't look around for a big church with an awesome special needs ministry. We had to hope our church would learn with us what James's needs would be and meet those needs. And they did! They created programs and outreaches to serve our family, like respite nights once a quarter, having a sensory-friendly room during the service for kids who weren't comfortable through the entire service, and buddies to help the kids who needed it in Sunday school and in all our summer activities. But these offerings blessed more than just our family. We reached new families, and saw parents respond to the gospel and get baptized. The church was a huge blessing to us in those early days and the years that followed.

We hear a lot about how churches can bless special needs families. But have you thought about all the ways special needs families bless the churches they attend? I can think of four big ways:

They remind them one size doesn't fit all (especially in children and teen ministry). When you start thinking outside the box for one student, you realize how many others don't fit in the box either. When I talk to churches about starting or expanding their ministries to special needs families, I often hear, "We have this one kid ..." but as we talk about solutions for him, we realize those solutions would work for even more kids!

Everyone can benefit from sensory toys or breaking complex lessons down to simple main ideas. When kids and teens consider the limitations their friends at church may have, it helps them grow to be more compassionate and empathetic. Paul says he becomes all things to all people to draw them to salvation. In 1 Corinthians 9:19 he writes, "For though I am free from all, I have made myself a servant to all, that I might win more of them" (1 Cor. 9:19). Special needs families remind churches they can be all things as well.

They model non-tradition methods of worship. In the church where we served in Pennsylvania, an eight-year-old girl with autism and her family sat in the front row so she could have room to dance. We were not a dancing church. But everyone loved watching her enjoy the music and praise God in her own way.

My friend Kathy writes about her adult son Joel, "It's a good thing that he loves to worship. And it's a God-thing to be part of a church where people smile when Joel wanders around the room during worship. Where the pastor sometimes invites him up to sing with the microphone. Where the congregation loves him and accepts him just as he is."

Greg Lucas writes about his son, "He cannot speak (although he can make plenty of noise) yet he is indispensable to the worship service. He constantly kicks the chair of the person in front of him, he claps during the quiet times and cannot sit still for five minutes, much less the length of a sermon. Yet he is indispensable to the church—indispensable to the body of Christ."

And Emily Colson says, "Most Sundays Max bounces so hard that one would expect him to go right through the wooden platform floor, dunk tank style. But he won't. Some of the men at church noticed the same risk. They got together one day and reinforced the floor where Max dances. It was months before anyone told me what the men had done."

Being able to walk around, clap when it's quiet, or bounce on the reinforced floor isn't the way everyone worships, but when everyone is able to worship in a way that matches their ability level, everyone benefits!

They comfort others with the comfort they have received. When we suffer, we look around for others who have experienced suffering. We don't want to hear false encouragement like, "God won't give you more than you can handle." That's simply not true. Abraham couldn't handle killing his son. Moses couldn't handle leading God's people across the Red Sea. Esther couldn't handle approaching the king to beg for her people's lives. Daniel couldn't handle the lions' den. They were all called to challenges they couldn't overcome on their own.

We do want to hear, "We know this is hard, we're sorry, and here's how we found hope." We want friends who will sit in the dust with me like Job's friends:

Now when Job's three friends heard of all this evil that had come upon him, they came each from his own place,

Eliphaz the Temanite, Bildad the Shuhite, and Zophar the Naamathite. They made an appointment together to come to show him sympathy and comfort him. And when they saw him from a distance, they did not recognize him. And they raised their voices and wept, and they tore their robes and sprinkled dust on their heads toward heaven. And they sat with him on the ground seven days and seven nights, and no one spoke a word to him, for they saw that his suffering was very great. — Job 2:11-13

The friends did a few things right: they came, they wept with him, and they sat. They shared in Job's suffering. They didn't think Job's bad luck would rub off on them. If you go to church each Sunday and everyone is smiling and saying they are fine, there's no room for hurting, suffering people. But when families like mine suffer and find joy in the midst of it, we can encourage other families to do the same.

They are frontline missionaries to an unreached people group—other special needs families. A special needs family is less likely to go to church than a typical family. What a great group to target, right? So how can we reach them? Use the special needs families as your missionaries! David Platt, President of the International Mission Board for the Southern Baptist Convention, says, "There are no unreached people in your office or neighborhood—because God has placed you there." And God has placed the special needs families who attend your church in a wide mission field!

I can't think of a group who needs the good news of the gospel more than special needs parents. They are the exact type of people Jesus ministered to when he was on earth. The hurting, the desperate, the weak, the angry, and so often, the hopeless.

And Jesus went throughout all the cities and villages, teaching in their synagogues and proclaiming the gospel of the kingdom and healing every disease and every affliction. When he saw the crowds, he had compassion for them, because they were harassed and helpless, like sheep without a shepherd. Then he said to his disciples, "The harvest is plentiful, but the laborers are few; therefore pray earnestly to the Lord of the harvest to send out laborers into his harvest." —Matthew 9:35-38

The special needs parents in your church can follow Jesus' example. They can look around and see their fellow special needs parents. They can have compassion on them. Pray to the Lord of the harvest to send out laborers and be ready to serve the families who visit!

I'm thankful for the ways our churches have blessed our family, and I hope the churches we have been a part of would say we blessed them as well. When special needs families are included in all aspects of church life, they are valuable members who bless as much as they are blessed.

• • •

AUSOME THOUGHTS

One of Merriam-Webster's definitions of the word "minister" is "agent." How exciting that God uses individuals with disabilities to be agents of change! They are changing church culture today to become more inclusive and loving, reflecting more of what Christ really intended for the New Testament church. This change ripples beyond the special needs community and touches every aspect of church life. We all benefit from these ausome ministers as they change the world, one church pew, one Sunday school class, one worship service at a time.

—Beth

chapter 13

Ausome Favor

by Laura Dodson

O N A SUPER WARM DAY in August, our family trotted off to our very first NFL football game. The ride to the stadium took over an hour and our sweet fun-loving Ryder would ask incessantly, "How long till we get there?" His voice growing more impatient the farther we drove. He was beside himself excited, yet the wait was almost unbearable. Ryder's love for the game, as they say, was priceless.

Let me set the stage for you. We are the Dodsons, the Fab 5 as we like to say. We have two teenage children, and Ryder our youngest has ausomely blessed our family. Ryder has a long list of special needs with autism being one of them. We find him to be an incredible blessing, uniquely created in God's own image. What happened this special day was nothing short of God's wonderful favor, an act of kindness beyond what we could ever have imagined.

We arrived at the stadium and waited for our very own personal family escort. I should tell you a few weeks prior I had asked my brother if he had any means of setting up something special for Ryder the day of our game. He had a few connections and was able to gain field passes for our family—the beginning of God's favor being given to Ryder that day.

We made the long haul to the field and saw the players were all in full gear beginning their pregame warmups! Ryder quickly became excited: hands flapping, clenched fists, the volume of his voice beginning to rise. He was over the moon at the simple sight of the field full of football players. Football, this is one of his loves, like the kind of love that you can't stop talking about, the kind of love that allows you to rattle off numbers and throw stats at any given moment. It was this kind of love that would allow the next few hours to be something we will never forget.

We stood on the out of bounds line (the line you not dare cross for fear of being taken off the field), and Ryder yelled out sweet sentiments to all the players, "Hi, TY," "Hi, Dwayne," "Good pass, buddy" ... This continued for a bit, all while his excitement level was rising. When Ryder gets excited, as with most kiddos on the spectrum, the world around them quickly fades away and nothing matters but the current moment of joy they find themselves in. He was quickly approaching that threshold! You know the one that can go so quickly south that you find yourself in a pile of blood, sweat, and tears?! Brad and I had discussed earlier in the day (like we do anytime we prepare for an outing) how it could go *really* good or it could go *really* bad—there's not a lot of room for gray.

But we continued to have God's favor. Things were going really well. Ryder's volume increased and players started to take notice. Dwayne #83 turned to Ryder, walked over to the line and went in for a high five, but Ryder would have no part of a simple high five and went straight for a hug! His personal space knows no boundaries! It was priceless. Later Dwayne would come back a second time for a quick game of pass with Ryder! He was ecstatic! So much so that he told this huge, kindhearted pro football player to "Go long!" And of course Dwayne did.

Brad and I looked at each other in disbelief. Our hearts connected knowing what a blessing this time was continuing to be for our precious son.

Ryder continued to make sure everyone knew he was still there, and God's favor continued to follow him. The crowd of people around us grew and I began to start all of the "autism-mom-thinking"—is he being too loud, is he making people uncomfortable, is he taking too much attention for himself—things that are always in the back of my mind. But it seemed for a while even for me, all of that faded away as we simply basked in his joy. A few minutes later we heard Ryder shouting out to Ty Hilton, "Hey, Ty, Hey, Hi, Ty, good job, Ty." Ty turned to do the typical wave, and I saw him have a total change of heart. He trotted over to Ryder and gave him a hug. He gave our sweet precious son, who adores him and his game, a hug. Ryder said, "I love you, Ty," and in return Ty said, "I love you too." Beautiful! That moment: amazing favor! God chose to use this completely innocent professional football player to bless our son. His act of kindness not only blessed Ryder but our entire family that day. A photographer had noticed the encounter ensuing and captured that sweet embrace in one perfect photo, one we will forever cherish. I am sure you can imagine the shrilling screams and non-stop jumping that would follow. After what seemed like a short fairy tale, we made our way to our seats. Because Ryder had depleted most of his energy (going from one emotion to the next, which happens so often), we only made it through half of the game. However the experience was enough to last a lifetime.

Of course, on our ride home we were all on cloud nine. The resounding words were, "Those NFL players took the time to come to Ryder out of the kindness of their hearts, and they blessed him more than they will ever know." We will never know if they could tell something was "different" or "unique" but what we can tell is that they chose to see Ryder's "ausomeness" and showed him favor that day.

Our oldest son happened to get photos and even was able to record the "Ty hug" on video, which was later played on local TV stations and ESPN's bleacher report, re-tweeted over three thousand times, and viewed more than half a million times on various social media platforms.

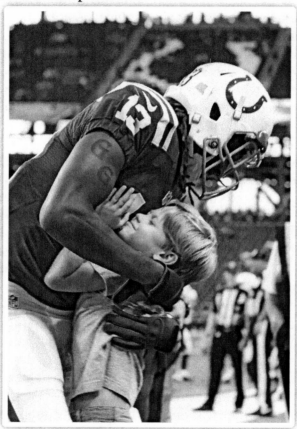

PHOTO CREDIT: ANGLE SIX

Later when the news stations aired the clip, we showed Ryder and he would simply say, "Ha, that's me." He knows no meaning of words like: famous, news, or ESPN. He had no idea the magnitude of the situation. It was simply a matter of the heart, and his heart was full. Our boy was shown much favor that special day and our family was implicitly blessed.

Moments like these make us forget all the hard days. It's with tears in my eyes as I write this months later that I am reminded of the ausome blessing we have been given. For so long we have lived in frantic mode, we have lived on high-alert, we have lived broken and desperate yet always prepared for what might come next. Over time you learn, you grow, you accept, you adapt. You give thanks for moments of favor. Moments like these allow us to put on our "gratitude glasses" and see things the way Ryder sees them, with joy, passion, and innocence. Ryder's emotions are raw, they are hard, but they are pure. There are good days, there are bad days, but we are so thankful for all of those days. I remember a time when we were told we may not take our son home—words that remind me I will continue to take all of those days: the good, the bad, and the ugly. And I will take them with a full heart, loving Ryder for who God created him to be, perfectly unique, unlike anyone else on the planet, unlike anyone else on the spectrum.

All of our children are his. "Every good and perfect gift is from above, coming down from the Father of Heavenly lights" (Jas. 2:17). We have all been given an ausome gift.

• • •

AUSOME THOUGHTS

Favor: to feel or show approval or preference for.

"You have granted me life and favor, and Your care has preserved my spirit" (Job 10:12). God favors all of his children, but it's those times that we see him working through a difficult situation, bringing about a miracle, answering a prayer in a big way that we truly know that his care has preserved our spirit. It's those times when he shows careful attention to the little details of our life—like giving a little boy a never-to-be-forgotten day on a football field—that make us know we live with ausome favor.

—Beth

Closing

S O YOU'VE MADE IT TO the end of this book. My prayer
is that by the time you reach this page, your heart will be
overflowing with thankfulness for the ausome blessing
in your life and that God will have given you a glimpse of the
amazing things he can do through disability.

I want to leave with one final account from scripture. Luke
10 has become a new favorite verse that I am praying over my
children.

*The Lord now chose seventy other disciples and sent them
on ahead in pairs to all the towns and villages he planned
to visit later. These were his instructions to them: "Plead
with the Lord of the harvest to send out more laborers to
help you, for the harvest is so plentiful and the workers so
few. Go now, and remember that I am sending you out as
lambs among wolves. Don't take any money with you, or a
beggar's bag, or even an extra pair of shoes. And don't waste
time along the way. Whenever you enter a home, give it
your blessing. If it is worthy of the blessing, the blessing will
stand; if not, the blessing will return to you. When you enter
a village, don't shift around from home to home, but stay in
one place, eating and drinking without question whatever
is set before you. And don't hesitate to accept hospitality, for
the workman is worthy of his wages! If a town welcomes you,*

> *follow these two rules: (1) Eat whatever is set before you. (2)*
> *Heal the sick; and as you heal them, say, 'The Kingdom of*
> *God is very near you now.'" — Luke 10:1-9, TLB*

Jesus is sending out disciples here while he is still on earth, sort of a test run, if you will, before he is not with them in the flesh. The disciples are to go from town to town ministering to people and healing the sick. Let's read on in this passage.

> *When the seventy disciples returned, they joyfully reported*
> *to him, "Even the demons obey us when we use your*
> *name." "Yes," he told them, "I saw Satan falling from heaven*
> *as a flash of lightning! And I have given you authority over*
> *all the power of the Enemy, and to walk among serpents*
> *and scorpions and to crush them. Nothing shall injure you!*
> *However, the important thing is not that demons obey you,*
> *but that your names are registered as citizens of heaven."*
> *Then he was filled with the joy of the Holy Spirit and said,*
> *"I praise you, O Father, Lord of heaven and earth, for hiding*
> *these things from the intellectuals and worldly wise and for*
> *revealing them to those who are as trusting as little children.*
> *Yes, thank you, Father, for that is the way you wanted it.*
> *Luke 10:17-21, TLB*

I love this account for so many reasons! Here these seventy disciples are returning and they are stoked! These disciples can't believe all the stuff they were able to do in Jesus' name. Jesus is rejoicing with them and tells them that he saw "Satan fall from heaven like lightning." Then Jesus goes on to have a praise party with the Father that these disciples obeyed and did mighty things in his name. Then he thanks the Father for hiding these things from the worldly wise and revealing them to the ones who are as trusting as little children, or I would say, ausomely blessed ones.

Here we see great and mighty things done by those with simple, childlike faith. I believe ausomely blessed individuals can easily take Jesus at his word, obey his commands, and do mighty things in his name. That seemed audacious to even type, but the scripture above proclaims it to be true. This is the way the Father wanted it, his truth revealed to those who innocently and easily believe what he says, and because they wholeheartedly believe what he says, it's easy to do what he commands.

One of my goals for this book was that it would be filled with scripture. Nothing can help us like the truth of God's Word. It is our unshakable foundation in times of trouble. Now that we have read the scripture in this book, it is my prayer that we too will simply and innocently take God at his word, boldly believe the promises he has given to us, and watch fear, worry, and the lies of the enemy fall from heaven like lightning. May the freedom of knowing we are ausomely blessed and living a life of favor cause us to go out and do mighty things in the name of Jesus!

Contributors

Terry and Karen Bishir are parents to four children; all are married and live in close proximity. They are blessed with eleven grandchildren, nine little girls and two little boys. Terry has pastored for forty years, almost thirty of those at the same church. Terry's passions include the study of God's Word, praying, and working physically on their home and wooded acreage. Karen splits her time between family; teaching middle and high school; directing the food service at the local school corporation; being involved in music and adult and children's ministries at their church; and walking/jogging with their dog Cooper.

Laura Dodson has been married to her highschool sweetheart for 18 years, and she grows more in love with him everyday. They live in a tiny little town called Sweetser. God has entrusted them with three of the most amazing littles! Carson, 17, is their oldest. He is a blonde-haired, blue-eyed, BIG-hearted child! Ireland, 15, their middle one is their only girl! She is a brown-haired beauty and has more will power and spirit than some adults! And their precious Ryder is 8. Laura loves being a mom, and her family brings her much joy. She puts her faith in Jesus and relies on Him daily! She loves all things health and fitness, being outdoors, running, coffee, and re-decorating their little home over and over! She works in direct sales and very much enjoys helping others reach their goals and find their potential, all while striving to better herself along the way.

Ryan Frank is a pastor, publisher, and an entrepreneur. He serves as the CEO of KidzMatter. Ryan and his wife, Beth, are the publishers of *KidzMatter Magazine*. He is also the Dean of Kidmin Academy. He is the author of *9 Things They Didn't Teach Me in College About Children's Ministry* (Standard), *Pulse* (KidzMatter), *Pulse 2* (KidzMatter), *Give Me Jesus* (Baker), and *The Volunteer Code* (The Leverage Group). Ryan and Beth live in Converse, Indiana with their three daughters. You can connect with Ryan at www.RyanFrank.com.

Dr. Stephen "Doc" Hunsley is the SOAR Special Needs Director and Pastor for Grace Church in Overland Park, Kansas. Doc started Grace Church's special needs ministry in 2011, helping it to become a hallmark ministry for the church. The SOAR (Special Opportunities, Abilities, and Relationships) special needs ministry serves over 650 individuals with special needs through weekend church programming, family support groups, and regular respite events. SOAR also has adult programming on the weekend, a VBS, and a Special Needs Day Camp in the summer. Doc founded and leads the Kansas City Special Needs Ministries Network for area church leaders. He is currently assisting over 150 churches locally and nationally to start a special needs ministry. Prior to serving as a special needs pastor, Doc was a children's pastor. Doc is a retired pediatrician while his wife Kay continues practicing pediatrics. They are proud parents to three beautiful children: Luke, Mark, and Sarah. The Hunsleys' middle child, Mark, is presently running the halls of heaven. During Mark's five-year earthly stay, he gave his family the opportunity to learn from and love a child with autism. You can follow SOAR Facebook at SoarSpecialNeedsMinistr yAtGraceChurch or connect with Doc on Twitter @DocHunsley or VisitGraceChurch.com/SOAR

Craig Johnson is the Director of Ministries at Lakewood Church, overseeing all pastoral ministries and staff; and the founder of Champions Club developmental centers for special needs, with over fifty across the world. He is the Executive Director of the nonprofit Champions Foundation, which provides education, spiritual growth, behavioral development, and services to individuals and families with special needs or who are medically fragile. Craig co-authored Champions Curriculum, the first full scope Christian Curriculum for Special Needs, and he is the author of *Lead Vertically: Inspire People to Volunteer and Build Great Teams That Last* and his new book *Unrehearsed Destiny: It's Intermission, Your Second Act Is Coming.* Craig and his wife of twenty-seven years, Samantha, have three children: Cory, Courtney, and Connor.

Sandra Peoples is a pastor's wife and mom to two boys. She's the author of Speechless: Finding God's Grace in My Son's Autism and Held: Learning to Live in God's Grip (a Bible study for special-needs parents). She and her family live outside of Houston, TX. You can connect with her at sandrapeoples.com

Barbara J. Newman is a school and church consultant for CLC Network. She is the author of several books and is a frequent national speaker at educational and ministry conferences, as well as churches. In addition to writing and speaking, Barbara enjoys working in her classroom at Zeeland Christian School. Learn more at clcnetwork.org.

Dr. Sandy Robinson has over thirty-three years of experience in public education. She has taught multiple subjects to students in grades five through twelve. She has also been a site administrator and the Director of Special Education in two different districts. Dr. Sandy has taught teacher preparation courses at California State University, Riverside. She has trained educators, administrators, and parents in the areas of positive behavior techniques, teaching and learning strategies, inclusion techniques, crisis intervention, and Special Education Law. She is an Inclusion Specialist. She brings her extensive experience in the field of special education to faith communities. Dr. Sandy is currently the Regional Director of Champions Club, an international ministry for students and adults with special needs and their families. In 2012, with the support of Pastor Craig Johnson and Covina Assembly of God Church, she developed and launched the first Champions Club outside of Lakewood Church. In 2014, Dr. Sandy and Mr. Craig Johnson wrote the first full scale curriculum for Champions (individuals with special needs). The curriculum encourages families to come to know God, love him, and to share his love with others. In 2017, they released a family devotional that provides families access to the curriculum. She has been married to her best friend for twenty-eight years. God has blessed them with two amazing daughters who love and serve God, and two pugs named Littleman and Tiny Dog. It is her desire to assist churches, of all denominations, to successfully include exceptional individuals and their families in all aspects of church life.

Emma Roudebush is a behavior consultant in central Indiana who has a love for God, chocolate, warm weather, and dogs. She holds degrees in both Elementary and Special Education and has a Masters in Applied Behavior Analysis with an emphasis on Autism. Being a stay at home mom and having the opportunity to work with a few children with special needs brings her inspiration. Emma's most cherished roles include being a wife to Nick, a farmer and artist, and a mother to two young children: Everhett and Marlene May.

Norma Puga served as an administrator in the legal field for over 15 years. She currently serves as Champions Club Director for Lakewood Church and Program Director for Champions Foundation. She helped launch the first Champions Club for special needs at Lakewood Church in 2009 which currently serves over 150 families. She has helped launch over 55 Champions Clubs around the world. Norma is an expert trainer, facilitator, and speaker for special needs. She is the mother of one son, Robert III. She has been married for 25 years to her husband, Robert II.

Beth Frank loves Jesus, her hubs, three girls, and thinking creatively. Looking at life as one God-sized adventure helps keep her sane as she tries to keep up with her husband Ryan and their three active girls. Beth is a co-founder of Kidmin Nation and, along with her husband Ryan, publishes *KidzMatter Magazine*. Along with being passionate about kidmin, Beth was inspired by her oldest daughter's autism diagnosis to start a ministry to special needs families called Ausomely Blessed. Most weeks you can find Beth playing taxi cab driver for her girls, drinking coffee, brainstorming new ideas in her shared office with Ryan, or doing ministry at her local church. Beth believes that all of life is sacred and enjoys serving Jesus along the way!